NUTRITION FOR SPORT

Wilf Paish

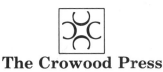

The Crowood Press

First published in 1990 by
The Crowood Press
Gipsy Lane, Swindon
Wiltshire SN2 6DQ

British Library Cataloguing in Publication Data

Paish, Wilf, *1932–*
    Nutrition for sport.
    1. Athletes Nutrition
    I. Title
    613.7

ISBN 1–85223–380–X

Whenever possible, measurements are given in both metric and
imperial units. However, this is not the case for very small weights
(for which no imperial equivalent is given) nor for units of energy
(when kilocalories only are given). If readers need to convert from
kilocalories to kilojoules, they should refer to Appendix 2, where
they will find a conversion table.

Typeset by Footnote Graphics, Warminster, Wilts
Printed and bound in Great Britain by BPCC Hazell Books Ltd, Aylesbury

261121

Contents

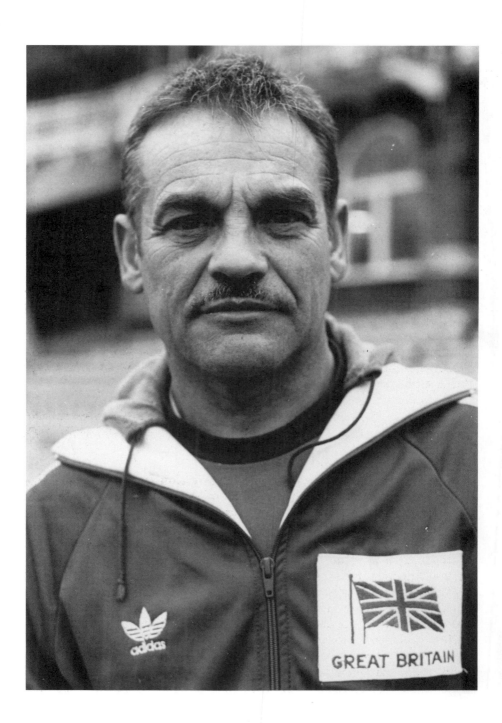

Forewords

Wilf Paish was my coach during the period leading up to the 1984 Olympic games in Los Angeles, where I won the gold medal in the javelin event. Wilf's general knowledge of what is required of an athlete, a coach and a sports scientist is recognised throughout the world and he is frequently asked to lecture, talk on television and so on about such diverse topics as diet and drugs.

Where there is as little as one per cent separating the gold medallist from the also-ran, future generations of world-record holders will have to look towards anything which is legal in order to help them tip the balance in their favour. Diet is a science which I am certain can do just that. During my entire career as an athlete and more recently as a television presenter, I have taken care of my personal appearance and I know that this is greatly affected by what I eat.

Tessa Sanderson MBE
Olympic gold medallist, javelin, 1984

Although Wilf Paish is best known as a leading athletics coach, his knowledge and interest covers a far wider range of sports. One of these is Rugby league, where he has been employed by Halifax Rugby League Football Club, in recent years one of the game's most successful clubs.

Wilf has brought to Rugby league important scientific principles, an analytical and an inquisitive approach that has helped in the game's tremendous recent developments. As Director of Coaching, I have used Wilf's expertise in the preparation of our senior professional international squad and on our coaching accreditation courses. Wilf has a unique ability to convert up-to-date scientific knowledge into easily understood terminology.

Recent improvements in Rugby league have been dramatic. The all-conquering 1982 Australian Kangaroos, who humiliated the British in an undefeated fifteen-match tour, caused a renaissance in coaching methods and playing standards which should begin to bear fruit in the 1990s.

The modern-day professional Rugby league player is a dedicated athlete, and aspiring young professionals are aware that only a total commitment to an intensive six-day-a-week training programme can guarantee success. Such intensive preparation cannot be achieved on two-star petrol. Correct eating habits and the maintenance of a proper diet are essential for success. I am therefore sure that Wilf's informative book, which is so easy to understand, will become an essential reference book for all Rugby league coaches and all ambitious players.

Phil Larder
Director of Coaching, The Rugby League

The world of sport has for too long been divided between the practitioners and the theorists. Rarely does one come across someone with a proven track record as a top international coach, who is also held in the highest regard by the academics, but Wilf Paish is such a person. Underlying his multi-sport background is his insistence on excellence in all that he does. One has to see Wilf in action to appreciate the quality of his work and his outstanding ability both to communicate and motivate.

Sports nutrition is an area in which Wilf Paish has become something of an authority and an area which has been given scant regard over the years. Too often the 'bit of what you fancy does you good' philosophy predominates. Only when all the areas that contribute to performance at any level are explored, does the value of nutrition become apparent. Whether in training or in competition, there is no doubt that the right fuel has to be in the tank! It is not just a question of adopting good habits, it is also a question of having the correct dietary intake according to the phase of the training or competition cycle. This book will undoubtedly provide much of the essential information needed. It is then up to each sportsperson to choose what he or she needs according to the guidelines given by Wilf.

Kevin Hickey MBE
British Olympic Boxing Coach

Acknowledgements

I would like to thank Anthony Franklin who kindly and skilfully produced the typescript, Eileen Langsley of Supersport Photographs who provided the photographic material, Margaret Still whose specialist knowledge of nutrition ensured accurate proof-reading during its many stages, to my family, who have had to make many sacrifices for my commitment to all aspects of sport which in turn has made this text possible. Finally, I would like to thank my wife who, as always, has been a tower of strength in helping me with the many facets of my work.

Introduction

How Good do You Want to Be?

Every day throughout the world, thousands upon thousands of people enjoy participating in various sports. At this level it does not matter unduly whether or not their levels of fitness or skill are high. However, at the other end of the scale, there are those ambitious individuals who wish to reach the highest pinnacles of sporting achievement. Within this group of people there are those who dedicate their whole lives to their

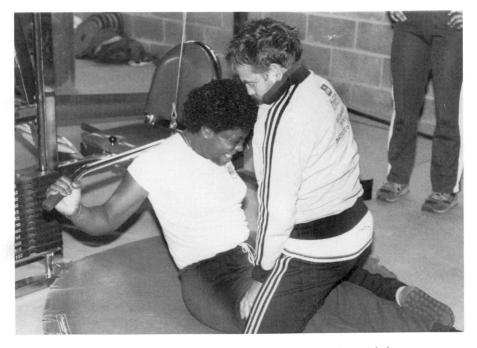

Fig 1   Tessa Sanderson undergoing some strenuous training with her coach before winning her gold medal in the 1984 Olympic games.

goal; there are others who undoubtedly have the ability but lack the commitment to achieve their far-sighted aims. Every day of my life I meet people in each of these categories. Quite early on in an athlete's career it is possible to detect the degree of commitment, skill and ability, and it is easy to predict their success. I also meet the excuse-orientated performer who is only too ready to admit that 'they would have been good if . . .' Frequently the 'if' means 'if they had the necessary commitment'.

I feel that anyone sufficiently interested to look deeply into nutrition as a means of enhancing performance has already made the necessary commitment to sporting excellence. To those about to make this decision I ask the question, 'How good do you want to be?' Think about it carefully, set your goals. Make a check-list of what you have to do to achieve these goals and read through these frequently as a reminder of the necessary commitment. Success in sport cannot be achieved without a sacrifice of some kind. In this case the sacrifice is of your time in order to pay attention to what is eaten, to resist the urge (especially in the hurly-burly of training and competing) of relying upon convenience foods and to pay special care to the energy balance; a few extra spare calories each day soon produces an inefficient overweight person.

While advice is available and certainly abounds within the pages of this text, only the individual can make the necessary commitment.

1

The Science of Sports Nutrition

This text is directed at the layman, the sportsperson and the coach and so it is not intended to delve too deeply into the scientific technicalities of the subject. However, a basic understanding of these is essential for a total appreciation of the contribution which nutritional therapy can make towards performance.

The sciences involved are: physiology (of cellular activity and of digestion and food absorption); biochemistry (of how food is transformed into energy to repair and maintain the sound and efficient morphological structure of the body); and chemistry (of the basic structure of essential nutrients).

Digestion

The food which we put into our mouths does not itself contribute directly to any of our functions. It all has to be processed and converted into chemicals which the cells of our body can then use. The actual process whereby the particles of food are turned into substances which the body can use is very complex. The act of swallowing a mouthful of food does not mean that the food is in the body; this does not occur until the converted substances appear in the blood or lymph streams so allowing them to be transported to the cells in all parts of the body.

The process of digestion starts in the mouth where the food is chewed (mastication), broken down into smaller particles and mixed with enzymes (which make the chemical process more efficient). The food is then swallowed. From the mouth the food enters the oesophagus where a peristaltic action transports it to the stomach, the main digestive organ. In the stomach, the food is mixed with gastric juices which contain enzymes capable of breaking down the food into the basic nutrients of carbohydrates and proteins; very little digestion of fats takes place in the

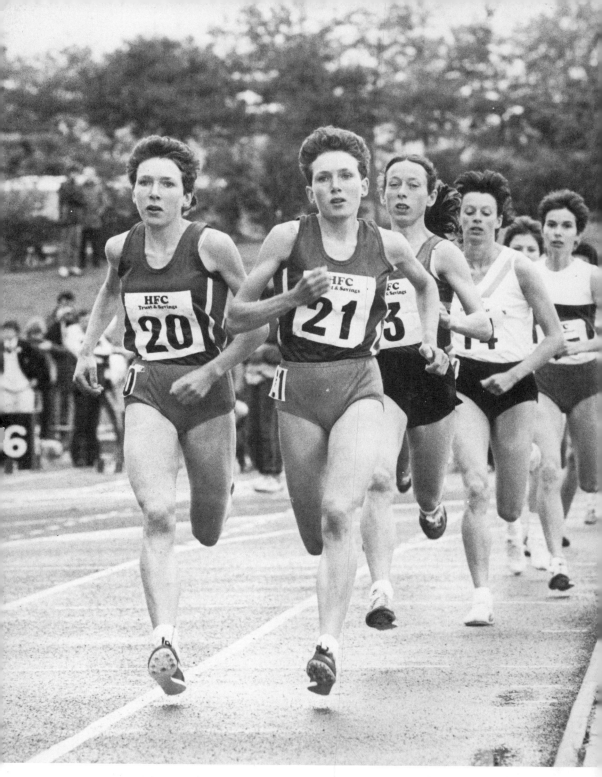

Fig 2   The very thin women of a typical middle-distance field.

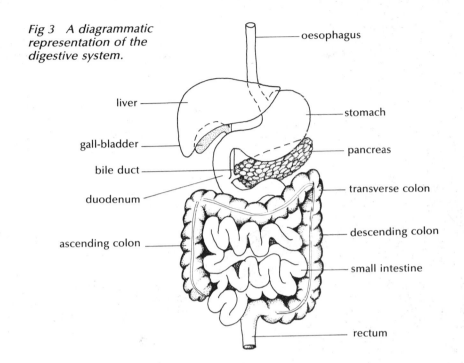

Fig 3 A diagrammatic representation of the digestive system.

oesophagus

liver

stomach

gall-bladder

pancreas

bile duct

duodenum

transverse colon

ascending colon

descending colon

small intestine

rectum

stomach. The food is churned and mixed in the stomach until it becomes a thin acidic liquid known as chyme. A similar peristaltic action draws the chyme to the pyloric end of the stomach from where it passes into the small intestine. It should be noted that very little absorption takes place in the stomach apart from alcohol and certain fast-acting drugs such as aspirin.

The small intestine is basically a coiled tube about eight metres in length, of which a small part is known as the duodenum – a very active digestive organ. On transit from the stomach to the small intestine, the food is acted upon by pancreatic juices (secreted by the pancreas which is situated behind the stomach). The pancreatic juices are very alkaline and so convert the chyme from its acidic state to a more neutral solution. The pancreatic juices contain special enzymes such as: trypsin, which helps the breakdown of proteins into their amino acid form; lypase, which has a basic action of converting fats to fatty acids; and amylase, which converts carbohydrates into simpler forms. The conversion in the small intestine is further complicated by intestinal juice which again converts the basic nutrients into forms which can be absorbed into the body. Apart from the specialised absorption aspect of the stomach as mentioned previously, all food absorption takes place once the food has left the duodenum.

While the liver is not considered part of the alimentary (digestive) mechanism, it does play an essential part in the utilisation, conversion and storage of our food and is a very active metabolic organ. At this stage of digestion it secretes a substance known as bile, which is stored in the gall-bladder. While bile does not contain any digestive enzymes it plays an important part in the absorption of fats as well as serving as a lubricant to aid the passing of substances through the intestine. More will be said about the liver later, particularly in its role of storing and converting energy products, for converting amino acids to carbohydrates, carbohydrates to fats and for the conversion of one amino acid to another.

Most of the conversion has been completed by the time the chyme leaves the small intestine. Carbohydrates are absorbed as monosaccharides, mainly by diffusion. Proteins are absorbed as amino acids either by absorption or by the specific active carrier system. Fats are absorbed as glycerol and fatty acids pass directly into the blood or lymphatic channels. Minerals are also absorbed into the system at this stage as is water, but by a more complicated process of osmosis.

The food finally passes into the large intestine where water is once again absorbed and the remainder, waste products, are expelled from the system in faeces. The whole complicated process is influenced directly by the various aspects of the nervous system and by the endocrine system through specialised hormones.

This brief introduction to digestion might stimulate further reading by those who wish to gain a deeper knowledge of the process. It is to be hoped that sufficient detail has been given to provide readers with a brief appreciation of the complicated process by which our food is converted into a usable state. The physiology of cellular activity is well beyond the scope of this text as the cells of the body are so specialised as regards the function which they perform that each aspect becomes a study in itself. However, it is important to remember that the activity of the cells requires energy, which they obtain from food. They are in a constant state of building up (anabolism) and breaking down (catabolism) the protein which is obtained from food.

The Chemistry of Food

Food can be broken down into three categories, each of which has numerous subcategories. The three main groups are basic nutrients, vitamins and minerals.

Basic Nutrients

The category of food known as basic nutrients is, in turn, made up of three subcategories, which are carbohydrates, fats and proteins.

Carbohydrates

As the word suggests carbohydrates are composed of carbon, hydrogen and oxygen. Carbohydrates can exist in the form of: monosaccharides – simple sugars – which include substances such as fructose and glucose (the latter being the form in which carbohydrate is present in the blood); disaccharides – double sugars – such as sucrose (cane sugar), lactose (milk sugar) and maltose (malt sugar); polysaccharides – multiple sugars – such as plant starch and glycogen (animal starch). The simple sugars are soluble in water whereas the compound sugars are not.

The body relies on carbohydrates for quick energy. The emphasis here is speed, for although both protein and fat can supply energy, they are by no means as quick or efficient. As carbohydrates readily release energy to the body a large part of an athlete's diet should be composed of carbohydrates. However, the body is only capable of storing about 2,500 kilocalories (kcal) of energy in this form. Exercise requiring more than this level of energy must be fuelled from other sources such as fats and proteins. Once carbohydrates have been depleted they are best replenished as quickly as possible. This (and carbohydrate loading) is discussed in Chapter 13.

It must be emphasised that carbohydrates are not vital to the functioning of the body since they do not produce any essential intermediary compounds, nor do they bind vitamins; they are simply very good at providing quick, efficient energy, largely because of the economic way in which they use oxygen for their metabolism. Excess carbohydrates are converted into fats to be distributed and stored about the body.

Fats

Fats (frequently referred to as lipids) are very similar in composition to carbohydrates except their ratio of oxygen to hydrogen is different. They offer a very high energy yield, somewhere in the region of two-and-a-half times that of carbohydrates, but they are uneconomical in their use of oxygen for metabolism.

Fats are compounds of a combination of triglycerides and glycerol and are converted into fatty acids for utilisation in the body. The fats which we eat come either from an animal or a vegetable source. Animal fats, which

17

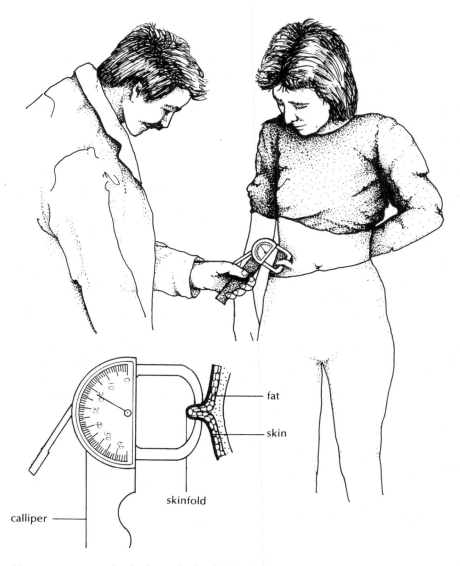

Fig 4 Estimating body fat with skinfold callipers.

are usually solid at room temperature, are termed saturated, referring to the fact that there are no available chemical bonds. The vegetable fats, mainly oils, are termed unsaturated, again for the same chemical reason (that chemical bonds are available).

Most western cultures eat far too many fats, particularly the saturated type, and there is sound evidence which links fats, especially cholesterol, with heart disease and obesity with certain forms of cancer. However, certain fats are essential to the body, in particular linolinic and linolenic acid. Fats are required to keep the skin in good condition, the kidneys working efficiently, to transport the fat-soluble vitamins (A, D, E and K), as a thermo-insulatory mechanism, for an efficient nervous system and in the production of certain hormones.

Fats, therefore, are most important to the body, but they must be taken in moderation. Unfortunately modern society has developed a taste for the hidden fats such as those found in crisps, roasted peanuts, biscuits, chocolate, pastry and such like, much of which form part of our social eating habits. In the diet fats also produce a post-meal euphoric effect mainly due to the slow transit through the gut, promoting the 'full' feeling.

When too much fat is consumed it is dispersed about the body in the form of adipose tissue, which produces the familiar bulges associated with those who over-indulge. Excess fat will make the body inefficient due to its effect upon the strength–weight ratio since, unlike muscle, fat is dead weight. Hence athletes should be concerned with their body-fat content; this can be measured by using skinfold callipers. Fit, young men will have a body-fat content of about eight to ten per cent, depending on the type of sport which they do, marathon runners being towards the lower end of this category. Women have a considerably higher percentage of fat than men. When the woman's body-fat content drops below 15 per cent amenorrhoea (abnormal absence of menstruation) is usually induced. This situation is evident in the current group of distance runners, who certainly look anorexic and exist very close to the borderline which divides health from illness. This group of women almost totally exclude fats from their diet, running the risk of kidney and hormone problems together with those associated with the lack of the fat-soluble vitamins, not to mention energy provision.

Proteins
Proteins are substances which contain nitrogen in addition to carbon and hydrogen. Indeed they are the body's single source of nitrogen, hence they are essential and must be included in our diet. A diet lacking in protein or sufficient energy to fuel daily life calls for the body to utilise its own protein from the cells and if the situation is prolonged, as in hunger strikes, death is certain to result. Proteins are essential because they are our cell-building and repairing agents. They have a profound effect upon

Food	Percentage
eggs	100
fish/meat	70
soya	69
milk	60
rice	56
corn	51

Fig 5   The relative availability of essential amino acids in certain foods. Eggs, the best source of these amino acids, are given a value of one hundred per cent, while corn can be seen to be roughly half as good a source. These figures are provided by the United Nations.

all aspects of homoeostasis, in particular the electrolyte balance and the existence and action of certain hormones. They have an energy-supplying function and are related to vitamin and enzyme activity – hence their contribution to a healthy life is, quite literally, vital.

Proteins are available to the body in the form of amino acids (small molecules which contain nitrogen). There are over twenty known amino acids, only eight of which are essential (EAA). As long as the body receives its supply of these eight it is capable of manufacturing the others. While most people can recognise the foods which contain carbohydrates or fats most would be hard pressed to decide which foods are high in protein. Like many aspects of nutrition the whole area is muddled with myths and fallacies. As long ago as 1956 the Food and Agricultural Organisation of the United Nations rated certain foods according to the availability and balance of essential amino acids. Eggs were found to be the best balanced and were given a rating of 100 per cent; other foods were rated on a decreasing percentage scale as shown in Fig 5.

It is also found that by combining certain types of these foods the percentage can be raised above 100 per cent. For example a mixture of egg and corn warranted a value of 125 per cent from the committee. Foods rich in protein come from two main sources: animal and vegetable foodstuffs. The animal proteins are often referred to as first class because they contain a good proportion of essential amino acids while vegetable proteins are frequently considered second class because they contain proportionately less. However, by mixing vegetable proteins alone the correct balance can still be achieved. Many dietary experts now go so far as to recommend taking more second-class proteins because they contain less fats than animal protein and are more likely to contain a better balance of minerals and vitamins.

Many sportsmen and women favour a diet containing a high protein content in the belief that it will help rebuild broken-down muscle cells. There does not seem to be a great deal of experimental evidence to support this although selected free-form amino acid supplements could provide stimulus for growth-hormone activity. The question of how much protein to consume will always remain a debatable point. Well-informed sources give values ranging from 25–150g (1–5oz.) per day. However, such values are vague since it must be related to lean body-mass. The generally accepted figure is in the region of 1g per kg of body-weight, with at least twice this for the growing child and power-based sportsmen and women.

Excess protein can be used for energy, in which case the nitrogen has to be excreted from the body. At certain times protein is indeed a valuable source of energy and more detail will be given regarding this in Chapter 5.

Some sportsmen and women are vegetarians and they, too, can have a perfectly healthy diet, especially if it contains cheese or milk. However, vegan diets, which are devoid of any animal products, can produce undesirable problems. It is sufficient to say that a great deal of thought should be given to vegetarian and vegan diets to ensure that they have the correct balance of amino acids from vegetable sources.

Vitamins

This is certainly the most controversial subject in the field of nutrition. It is a field with the most ardent supporters, including highly qualified doctors who use vitamin therapy in the treatment of a number of serious illnesses, and with the most ardent detractors, who condemn them outright and suggest that they do nothing more than produce expensive urine. While the study of vitamins has been in vogue now for over a century, few people know their precise role in the normal functioning of the body. What most researchers can prove is that the body cannot function normally and efficiently without them. They must be regarded as the catalysts of nutritional chemistry making any such actions within the body more efficient. Vitamins have a close interaction in the body, the presence of one being essential to the correct functioning of another. The body cannot manufacture vitamins and while they are required in only small amounts our only source is the food which we eat.

Vitamins are either fat soluble (A, D, E and K) or water soluble (B and C). If fat-soluble vitamins are taken in excess they could prove toxic since they are stored in the body. Water-soluble vitamins are less easily stored in the body and are fairly rapidly excreted in the urine. They are less stable than their fat-soluble counterparts and so their presence is depleted by cooking, freezing, storage, transport and other similar activities. While vitamin deficiency could have a very adverse effect upon the efficient functioning of the body (these days most sportsmen and women supplement them as an added precautionary measure), it still remains that the best insurance policy against any deficiency is to eat a wide variety of fresh fruit and vegetables. It is my established belief that if sportsmen and women eat a selection of two root vegetables, two green vegetables and at least two pieces of fruit every day, they are well on their way to a balanced vitamin intake.

Certain drugs, in particular the 'wide-spectrum' antibiotics, have a devastating effect upon a number of vitamins, especially the B group (this occurs notably in the gut). At this stage it is desirable to identify the vitamins, what effects their presence or absence has on the body and their main sources in the food which we eat.

The chart on pages 62 and 63 gives more specialised information on vitamins and should be used in conjunction with the following general information.

Vitamin A
The true vitamin A is only found in animal foods, but provitamin A, or carotene, is found in green vegetables and carrots. Low-fat dairy products and low-fat spreads contain little or no vitamin A, nor is it found in white meat, fish and white vegetables. It is stable to heat, but is affected by light and oxygen, hence storage in the light will affect its properties.

Vitamin B_1
This vitamin is added to most bread and cereals in the UK. It is readily destroyed by cooking and freezing. Most foods have some vitamin B_1 in them, although refined starches, sugar and alcohol contain very little.

Vitamin B_2
Very similar in composition to B_1. However, it is fairly stable in heat so little is lost in cooking. It is destroyed by ultra-violet rays so once gathered it should be kept out of the sunlight.

Vitamin B_3 (Niacin)
Niacin can be made from the amino acid tryptophan. While niacin is found in most foods it is absent in alcohol and refined foods. It is very stable in cooking.

Vitamin B$_6$ (Pyridoxine)
The need for this vitamin is increased for those not on a high-protein diet. It is most unstable in water, especially during cooking.

Vitamin B$_7$ (Choline)
Produced in the body from protein, it is important in the function of lecithin (*see* page 58).

Vitamin B$_{12}$ (Cyanocobalamin)
There is very little of this vitamin in plant food, hence vegans must supplement their diet to obtain it. While it is stable in cooking there is some leakage into the water.

Folic Acid
Much of its value is lost in cooking and other forms of preparation. It occurs in vegetables, pulses and whole-wheat products.

Biotin
Common in most foods, it can also be manufactured in the intestine. It is unaffected by processing and cooking.

Vitamin C
This is only really available in any quantity in vegetables and fruit. It is very vulnerable to cooking and preserving when most of its value is lost.

Vitamin D
This is only present in a few foods, its main source being fish oil. Removing fat from the food, such as by grilling, frequently reduces the value of this vitamin.

Minerals

Most people confuse the actions of minerals and vitamins, mistakenly believing them to be the same. While to a degree this might be true in that they both contribute to a healthy life, it is far from the truth in terms of their action upon the bodily systems. Basically, the minerals within the body can be divided into two groups. The first group determines the very delicate balance of cellular fluids and is frequently referred to as electrolytes. The second group has an effect upon the morphological structure of the body, such as the bones and teeth. There is also a third group which contributes to a number of enzyme reactions which in turn influence a person's total well-being. The last group contains those minerals known as trace elements.

The Electrolyte Balance

All of the cells in our body are bathed in cellular fluid. This environment must be kept stable, yet the concentration of the fluid is constantly changing. Homoeostasis is ensured by the minerals consumed in our food being called upon to keep the status quo. These minerals include sodium, potassium and chlorides. However, the total action of the fluid balance is a very complicated one and far beyond the scope of this text.

Morphological Minerals

Calcium is the most abundant mineral in the body since our bones and teeth are mainly composed of this mineral. Our bones are constantly being broken down and rebuilt, hence the body's need for this mineral. If the bones are not kept in a constant state of repair they become brittle and more susceptible to cracking or even fracturing. Calcium is also required for the rhythmic contraction of both cardiac and skeletal muscle. A deficiency can cause a spontaneous twitch, when certain muscles go into involuntary contractions.

The normal assimilation of phosphorus and protein is dependent upon calcium. It can be stored in the body (in particular in the gut) where it binds itself with excess fat for deposit. This mineral is ever-present in dairy products and green, leafy vegetables. However, there is one precaution to be borne in mind; it competes with magnesium for absorption from the gut hence at times, and in particular during hot weather when magnesium and calcium supplementation might be necessary, this factor must be regarded. Calcium cannot be absorbed without vitamin D, thus giving further evidence of the interdependence of certain vitamins and minerals.

Magnesium interacts closely with the fluid-balancing minerals, sodium and chlorides. It is well documented that where such an imbalance arises, muscle cramp results. There cannot be a sportsperson who has not suffered from this almost paralysing condition. It is frequently associated with exercise in hot climates and some athletes resort to salt-tablet therapy.

Iron

This mineral plays an essential role in the transportation of oxygen. Iron is the colouring pigment of haemoglobin, to which oxygen attaches itself so that it can be transported to the active tissues for chemical respiration. A shortage of iron leads to a condition known as anaemia, whereby the blood has a reduced capacity to carry oxygen and produces the symptoms of fatigue and breathlessness during physical exertion. It is a symptom readily recognised in the pallor of the skin; particularly notice-able is the colour of the eyelids. It is a condition which most adult women experience more than men due to their monthly menstrual losses. While a number of top sportswomen, through heavy training loads and a reduction in body fat, induce a condition of amenorrhoea, anaemia is a condition that must not go untreated. Indeed many sportswomen take regular doses of iron preparation, such as ferrograd C, to ensure against this condition. It must be noted that iron cannot be absorbed without the presence of vitamin C, so where the iron preparation does not contain vitamin C, ascorbic acid supplementation must accompany it. Excessive iron intake can produce the adverse reaction of vomiting and diarrhoea, but intake would have to be very substantial to produce this condition. Foods such as offal, green vegetables (including watercress and spinach) are very rich in this mineral and so should be regularly included in the diet.

Trace Elements

These include such substances as chromium, nickel, tin, vanadium, silicon and fluorides, all of which are essential for healthy life. Their action is not fully understood and is constantly being researched by those working in the field of nutritional therapy. A lengthy discussion on this aspect of nutrition is too complex for a work of this nature.

Dietary Fibres

These are substances which pass through the digestive system without being absorbed, but are nevertheless essential for the physical well-being of the body. The fibres are commonly referred to as roughage and there are many diets which include a high proportion of fibre. Most first-world countries tend to eat too much of the refined foods in which the fibre content is extremely low. Ultimately this can cause terminal infections of the gut. Researchers have frequently found that people from nations which include a high proportion of fibre in their diet have a higher resistance level to cancer and similar conditions which infect the intestines.

Dietary fibres can almost be considered as the scouring pad of the intestine. They tend to absorb and collect unwanted materials such as the acid bile which if left in the system would cause unpleasant side-effects. Fibre also tends to increase the water content of the stool, acting as a dilutant of materials in the colon and large intestine, again avoiding a situation that could produce discomfort.

Water/Fluids

Fluids are always important to the functioning of the body and even more so when the body is involved in exercise. Minute changes in the fluid structure of the body can have a disastrous effect upon its performance. It is possible to survive for several weeks without food but only a few days without water.

Fluids play a vital role in homoeostasis, be it the external or the internal environment of the body which causes the imbalance and which must be quickly redressed. The cells of our body are bathed in fluid and because of constant cellular activity the chemical composition of this fluid is continually undergoing change. Fluids carry nutrients, transport the by-products of metabolism and can help to regulate temperature. Such a situation calls for the body to secrete fluid in an attempt to maintain an equilibrium, but this equilibrium is only possible when the liquid is quickly replaced. If the fluid is not replaced then dehydration will result. Without doubt the finest replacement fluid is water although special electrolyte replacement drinks are available for specific situations; however, extra care must be taken to make sure that replacement drinks are necessary. Drinks, such as those saturated with glucose, can trigger a response from the body which is the reverse of the intended response. No such adverse reaction would be forthcoming if the replacement fluid is water. Any alcoholic drink actually causes dehydration and so should be avoided when fluids are needed.

The exercising body needs fluid, little and often, before, during and after activity. If this becomes a regular pattern – a habit – for the sportsperson, the symptoms of dehydration should never be experienced.

The problem with this introductory chapter has been what to omit, not what to include. It is my intention to give sufficient insight into the science of nutrition to understand what is to follow. I hope this goal has been achieved.

2

The Metabolism

A text of this nature must always try to answer the basic questions of why, what, how and when. Each of these basic questions could be directed at more than one area of nutrition. For example, the 'how' question could be directed at 'How can nutritional science be used to enhance performance?' or, 'How much do we need to eat?' Hopefully, this chapter will go a long way towards answering both questions. It will involve the study of energy: how the body gets energy from the food we eat; how the body utilises and turns it into physical activity; how energy is measured and the need to understand the energy balance.

The study of nutrition embraces a number of other sciences such as physics, biology, physiology and chemistry. The pure physicist recognises energy as the capacity to do work. This is basically what a person does in sport, turning one form of energy into another form to produce work. However, there must be energy there to start with, so where does the basic 'cycle' start? The source of all energy is the sun. The radiant energy produced by the sun is used in conjunction with chlorophyll to produce food which we can either eat directly, through vegetables, or intermediately, through animal products. In this case the animal has converted the stored vegetable energy into another store which human beings capitalise on when they eat animal products. So, man relies upon photosynthesis to obtain the energy which is stored in the chemical bond of the glucose module. The energy stored in the glucose module can be liberated by oxidation and used to do work and to produce heat. It is the linking of the fields of dynamics and thermodynamics which provide us with the units used in nutrition. The basic unit of energy used by the current researchers is the joule (J) and the kilojoule (kJ). However, it will take a very long time for nutritionists, researchers and writers to convert from the more common unit of the calorie and the kilocalorie. (Common usage uses calories when, technically, kilocalories are intended. In this book, kilocalories are used throughout rather than the erroneous calories.)

To put these units into perspective, the human body, as a result of the cells using energy, radiates heat at the rate of approximately one

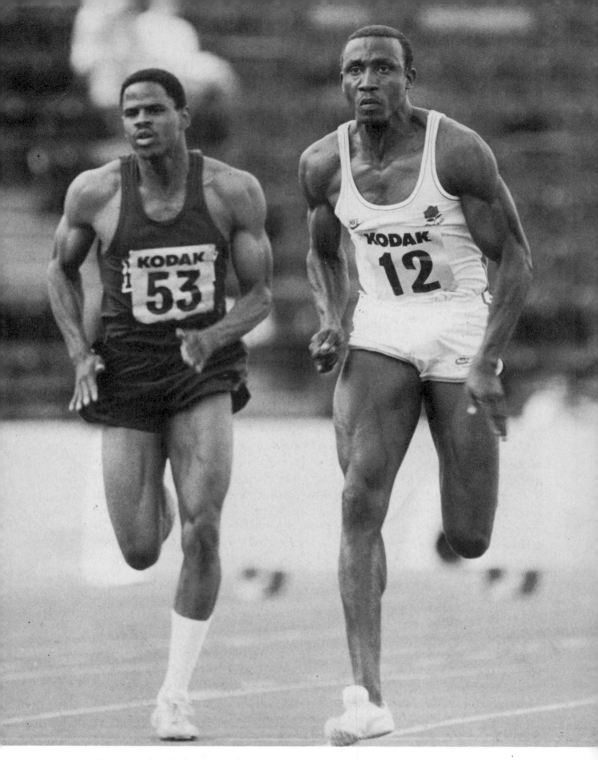

Fig 6   Linford Christie, who trains for several hours each day, but competes for just a few seconds.

kilocalorie (kcal) per minute. The output of a one kilowatt (kW) electric fire is about fourteen kilocalories per minute, hence the feeling of warmth when in a crowded room. These two units used in the field of nutrition to measure energy can be converted from one to the other. There are 4.186 kJ to each kilocalorie, hence to convert kilocalories to kilojoules a quick division by 4.2 will provide the approximate answer. An accurate conversion table is given on page 122.

When the human body converts the chemical energy in foods it does so through an oxidation process which is made possible only by intricate enzyme activity. Without this the energy in food could not be released at body temperature, but even with this enzyme activity the foods are not completely burnt in terms of thermodynamics. However, such a process can be performed in the laboratory and it is this complete process which can establish a heat value for any particular type of food. The apparatus for determining this value is known as the Bomb calorimeter. In this a particular food is mixed with oxygen at a very high pressure, then ignited with an electric spark and the resulting heat produced is accurately measured. With this method it can be calculated that each gram of carbohydrate yields 4.1kcal of energy, protein 5.6kcal and fats 9.3kcal.

However, the human body is not as efficient as the laboratory process, and so these figures cannot be used in our calculations. This inefficiency arises because digestion is not complete and a proportion of the energy in food is excreted. This is particularly the case with protein, of which a relatively large amount of the energy content is lost in the urine (somewhere in the region of eight per cent). The human system is very efficient at digesting carbohydrates with only a loss of about one per cent. The recalculated figures therefore become:

carbohydrates	4kcal/g
proteins	4kcal/g
fats	9kcal/g

Many of the texts on nutrition contain tables of food which give the food's energy equivalent and then break it down into the basic food categories. While such tables do serve as a guide they cannot be totally accurate and so must be treated with caution. It is suggested that they are little more than eighty or ninety per cent accurate, thus making nutrition not quite as exact a science as physics, for example.

Food	Energy (kcal)	Water (g)	Protein (g)	Fats (g)	Carbohydrates (g)
bread	243	38.3	7.8	1.4	52.7
milk	66	87.0	3.4	3.7	4.8
butter	793	13.9	0.4	85.1	slight
cheese	425	37.0	25.4	34.5	slight
potatoes (raw)	70	80.0	2.5	slight	15.9
cabbage (raw)	20	78.0	1.3	slight	1.3
peas (cooked)	80	72.0	6.0	slight	16.0
meat	270	56.0	20.0	20.0	0
fish	17.5	65.0	20.0	8.3	3.6
apples	47	84.1	0.3	slight	12.2
bananas	60	60.0	0.7	slight	14.0
tomatoes	20	75.0	1.0	slight	5.8
cucumber	15	80.0	0.5	slight	5.2

Fig 7   Common foods and their main nutrient content.

For life to be sustained, energy degradation must take place. The rate of degradation varies considerably from person to person and from moment to moment. However, there are certain standardised situations which have a major influence, which are: weight; height; age; and sex. All of these considerably influence the basal rate of a person, which is the rate of energy degradation of a person at rest, perhaps a period of twenty-four hours' bed rest. Physical work also has a major influence on the basal rate, which can be increased two- or even three-fold during bouts of very strenuous activity.

It is possible to calculate with some degree of accuracy the amount of energy a person will expend in a twenty-four-hour period. Researchers have arrived at energy values for all our daily chores, such as dressing, sitting still and so on, for all of our work activities, whether as a carpenter, electrician or whatever, and for all our enjoyment-based activity. With this in mind one can then arrive at a formula to calculate daily expenditure of energy:

basal rate + chores + work + enjoyment activity

This will be discussed in greater detail when specific sport-related consider-ations are examined in Chapters 8–12. For the time being, it is sufficient to say that it is possible to make calculations for the average person based on the above information. The generally accepted norm for the UK is a daily energy of 3,000kcal, but this must be regarded as very approximate.

These basic calculations are sufficient for a consideration of an aspect of life which is essential for physical well-being: the energy balance. For example, the average person should take in just sufficient food energy to balance the 3,000kcal expended through daily activities. If a person eats more in terms of energy than is required to maintain a balance, the energy is converted into fat and stored about the body. Ultimately, if this situation is maintained the result is obesity. On the other hand, if a person eats less than is required, weight loss is experienced and, ultimately, death will occur.

While there are only minor fluctuations of body-weight over a day, the cumulative affect over a period of fifty years would prove debilitating – just one extra potato crisp per day could produce a person many pounds overweight. It is interesting to note that over the period of adult life the average person gains 12kg (26lb) in weight, yet the average ingestion of food is about 20,000kg (20 tons) over the same period.

So, how much does the average person need to eat? The UK recommended diet is shown in Fig 8. This shows that a person should ideally eat food which provides the total amount of kilocalories and is comprised of the correct proportions of the basic nutrients. However, such a situation would be impossible for the average person to monitor and so the simple answer is that one should eat daily from a wide variety of food and then carefully monitor body-weight, taking care to avoid anything other than minor fluctuations by changing the content of the diet.

Nutrients	Weight (g)	Energy (kcal)	Percentage of energy requirement
protein	86	350	11
fats	141	1,250	39
carbohydrates	414	1,590	50
		3,190	

Fig 8   This table shows the UK recommendation for the average person's diet per day.

The discussion to date has been totally influenced by energy degradation; in basic terms we have only covered half of metabolism. The question of how the body produces energy from food still needs to be answered. However, there has to be a store of energy before it can be degraded. The production of this store is known as chemical metabolism. In order to function, the cells of the body require a high-energy

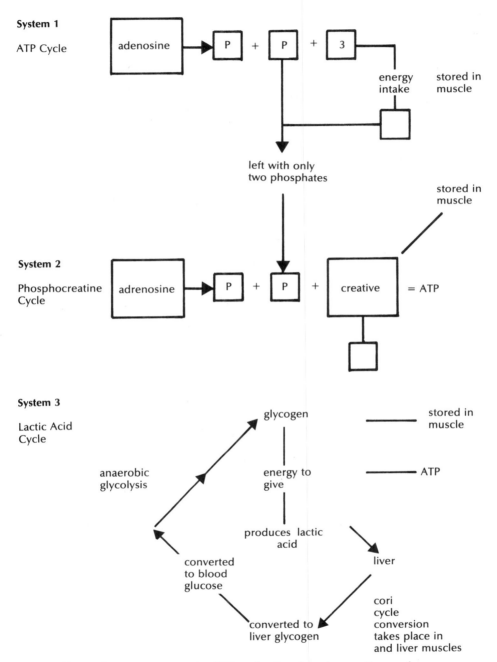

System 1

ATP Cycle

adenosine → P + P + 3

energy   stored in
intake   muscle

left with only
two phosphates

stored in
muscle

System 2

Phosphocreatine
Cycle

adrenosine → P + P + creative = ATP

System 3

Lactic Acid
Cycle

glycogen   ————   stored in
muscle

anaerobic
glycolysis

energy to
give   ———— ATP

produces lactic
acid

liver

converted
to blood
glucose

converted to
liver glycogen

cori
cycle
conversion
takes place in
and liver muscles

*Fig 9   Energy systems: 1   ATP cycle; 2   phosphocreatine cycle;
3   lactic acid cycle (anaerobic glycolysis); 4   aerobic cycle.*

System 4

Aerobic Cycle

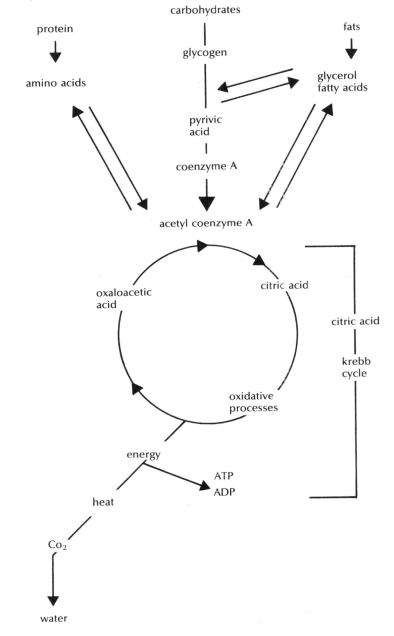

phosphate, called adenosine triphosphate (ATP). The body must have a constant supply of this substance and the cyclic way in which the body is assured this supply is known as the energy system. Which cycle the body uses depends upon the intensity of the demand for energy.

The co-ordinator or conductor of the 'metabolic orchestra' is the liver. All the end-products of digestion which are used in the production of energy pass through the liver, where they can be stored or directed to the cells requiring energy. Each of the basic nutrients are metabolised in a different way. Carbohydrates are absorbed from the alimentary canal in the form of fructose, galactose or glucose. These are converted in the liver to glycogen, which is then absorbed into the blood as blood glucose, transported to the muscles and converted into muscle glycogen, where it is then converted again in the mitochondria to ATP. The exact sequence of events depends upon whether sufficient oxygen is available to complete the metabolism. With sufficient oxygen the process is termed aerobic and when combustion is forced to take place in the absence of oxygen the term used is anaerobic.

In the presence of oxygen, glycogen is broken down into ATP and its by-products; pyruvic acid, carbon dioxide and water. In this situation each molecule of glycogen yields thirty-eight molecules of ATP. In the absence of oxygen, glycogen is still oxidised but the by-product is a paralysing substance known as lactic acid. In this anaerobic cycle each molecule of glycogen produces only two molecules of ATP. Indeed, the anaerobic system is only capable of providing energy for a very restricted period of time, in the region of three to five seconds. Once the ATP is broken down (by the removal of the phosphate to liberate energy) the system is left with a substance known as adenosine diphosphate (ADP). If there were no means of utilising ADP for energy production, activity would have to cease as soon as the supply of ATP was exhausted. However, the muscle also has a store of a substance known as creatine phosphate (or phosphocreatine, PC), which has a single phosphate bond. This combines with the remaining diphosphates to produce a further supply of ATP. To assure a further supply of energy, the lactic acid enters the blood stream and is transported to the liver which in turn converts the lactic acid to liver glycogen; this then enters the bloodstream as blood glucose and in the muscle is converted again into muscle glycogen, so extending the availability of energy. Unfortunately, not all of the lactic acid is converted in the liver; some remains in the system and this starts to accumulate. Eventually, this becomes intolerable whereupon exercise must cease.

The body has three levels of producing anaerobic energy:

1. Glycogen is stored in the muscle. Enzyme activity causes energy release leaving a by-product of ADP.
2. Phosphocreatine, stored in the cells, can be used to reconstitute ATP from ADP.

Both of these mechanisms are short-lived and provide a total of less than ten seconds' energy supply.

3. Glycogen is resynthesised from lactic acid as part of the function of the CORI cycle and is returned to the active muscles. This third level has a slightly extended life but again is subject to severe limitations.

If all three levels are depleted, the state of high activity has to be reduced in order to allow the aerobic system to take over. To summarise, the immediate source of energy for muscular contraction is ATP and it is vital that this compound is continuously resynthesised. As its supply is very limited its immediate form of resynthesis is by splitting creatine phosphate, of which there is a limited store in the muscles and continuing with ADP. These phosphogens must be replaced and this can be achieved by the combustion of food or by glycolysis, in which glycogen is broken down to form lactic acid. The lactic acid can be resynthesised back to glycogen by utilising energy from food combustion. In these reactions there are three energy-producing systems which are: food combustion; splitting of phosphogens; and glycolysis. The energy-absorbing systems are phosphogen resynthesis and glycogen reconstitution.

The understanding of energy systems is relatively new to sport and fresh evidence arrives daily to shed more light on how the body can sustain relatively long periods of high activity and how all of our basic nutrients contribute to this supply of energy. It is a field which has captured the imagination of coaches, who experiment with different training programmes in an attempt to stimulate a particular energy system, so enhancing its contribution to the total energy cycle.

So far we have only discussed energy and the production of energy, and intimated that the energy is utilised both in the process of living and in sporting activities. However, it must be accepted that an individual's metabolic rate is not constant. There are a number of both extrinsic and intrinsic functions which influence it. This is largely controlled by the activity of certain hormones. This field is beyond the scope of this text, but it is opportune now to discuss those personal factors which the nutritionist can take into consideration and make allowances for when calculating an individual's total requirement for energy.

Size

Size has the most significant effect upon energy requirements. Unfortunately, it is a factor which is constantly ignored when planning menus and training programmes for the large field eventer or Rugby forward, in particular. It can be best understood by using some of the information listed earlier in this chapter. Calculations can be related to the physical property of work, which is defined as force × distance. Compare two different people who raise their body-weight up a set of steps 1m (3ft) high; person A weighs 60kg (132lb) and person B 90kg (198lb).

Person A performs 60kg × 1m (132lb × 3ft) = 60 (396)
Person B performs 90kg × 1m (198lb × 3ft) = 90 (594)

To perform this activity, person B must exert fifty per cent more energy than person A. This example would also be used to illustrate the training stress upon two Rugby players. A would be a typical back player, while B would be characteristic of a forward. During running activities the forward would have to perform fifty per cent more effort, but is unlikely to have a fifty per cent greater reserve of energy. This illustrates the importance of training for specific sports. It also illustrates the stress which could be placed upon the body through obesity.

| Weight | | Energy expenditure per day |
(kg)	(lb)	(kcal)
	Men	
64	140	1,550
73	160	1,640
82	180	1,730
91	200	1,815
100	220	1,900
	Women	
45	100	1,225
54	120	1,320
64	140	1,400
73	160	1,485
82	180	1,575

Fig 10   Differing basal rates for people of different body-weights.

From the information in Fig 10 it can be deduced that there is a marked difference in basal rate between a person weighing 64kg (140lb) and a person weighing 100kg (220lb). Indeed, the difference in energy expenditure for twenty-four hours of bed rest is 350kcal. There is a also a slight gender difference of something in excess of 100kcal.

Height

Height makes only a very marginal difference to basal rates, although it should be regarded if highly accurate calculations are required. Fig 10 assumes an average height of 178cm (5ft 10in) for men and 168cm (5ft 6in) for women. A figure of 20kcal should be added for every 2.5cm (1in) above this height and subtracted for every 2.5cm (1in) below this height.

Age

Research has indicated that the basal metabolic rate decreases with age. Fig 10, standardised with reference to height, is also standardised so far as age is concerned, the norm being twenty-five years. For every ten years above this age, the energy requirements should be reduced by 4 per cent.

Climate

Everyone has experienced the effects of climate and of environment upon their appetites, albeit quite subjectively. While on a seaside holiday, irrespective of activity, or when outside on a cold day, the appetite naturally increases. On a hot, humid day the reverse effect is noticed. It is hard to pin-point the precise nature of the change. It is possible that on a cold day the basal metabolic rate is speeded up (in extreme cases shivering causes large muscle groups to adopt a spontaneous form of activity) in an attempt to keep the body warm by generating heat. Protective clothing increases weight, restricts movement and so calls for a greater muscular effort, with an associated increase in energy expenditure. The reverse may also be the case when the environment becomes warmer. However, researchers have found that when exercising, in a warm environment, the demand for oxygen can increase by approximately ten per cent.

A degree of acclimatisation can usually be achieved, hence the need for sportspeople to consider this option when activity is contemplated in a different environment. However, any degree of acclimatisation – when compared with those nurtured in the different environment – can only be partial. Hence the native has an innate advantage over the visitor.

Everyday Chores and Work

So far, we have only really dealt with the calculation of the basal rate, that is the energy required to fuel the internal workings of the body, to maintain the beating of the heart, the ventilation of the lungs, the passage of food during alimentation, the excretion of waste products and the synthesis of new tissue while at rest. However, only the unfortunate are totally confined to bed; all others, to a varying degree, must be active in order to lead a normal life. There are such chores as washing, dressing, walking up and downstairs, standing, sitting, eating, bed-making and so on, indeed, a whole host of activities all of which require considerably more energy than bed rest. Researchers have calculated the approximate energy costs of such activities. Fig 11 shows examples of the energy requirements for such activities.

Activity	kcal/kg/hr
sitting still	1.43
standing	1.50
walking	2.86
dressing/undressing	1.69
light work	2.00
moderate work	5.70
heavy occupational work	7.50

Fig 11   The energy costs of various routine activities.

In this situation it is always difficult to decide where a person's daily chores end and his or her occupation starts. For example, a person might have to sit still for long periods as part of their job of work. Also, it is very hard for the average person to be precise in the recording of all their chores, the time taken on each, the type of movement involved in transferring from one activity to another. This would place everyone in a laboratory-type situation, surrounded by stop-watches and other monitoring devices. The careful evaluation of such figures, however, even for serious sportspeople, is neither necessary nor desirable. To allow for general calculations, researchers have calculated a percentage allowance above the basal rate for most work situations, as shown in Fig 12.

Activity	Percentage above basal rate
quiet sitting	30
light activity (office work)	50
moderate activity (housework)	70
heavy occupational work	100

Fig 12   The percentage allowance above the basal rate for work situations.

Using Fig 12, the following calculations will serve as an example to illustrate the complete energy requirements before any adjustments are made for sport.

Energy required = basal rate + chores + occupational allowance

1. Female, 25 years old
   Height: 168cm (5ft 6in)
   Weight: 64kg (140lb)
   Occupation: typist

Basal rate	1,400kcal
Occupation + chores allowance (=50%)	700kcal
Total (per day)	2,100kcal

2. Male, 35 years old
   Height: 178cm (5ft 10in)
   Weight: 82kg (180lb)
   Occupation: labourer

Basal rate (=1,730kcal − 4% age allowance)	1,661kcal
Occupation + chores allowance (=100%)	1,661kcal
Total (per day)	3,322kcal

To conclude by returning to the energy balance hypothesis; for a healthy lifestyle it is important that people do not carry around with them excess fat. The obese person places a considerable stress upon the physiological system, in particular the heart and respiratory organs. Hence, the energy balance is critical especially during those years of adulthood before the natural process of old age starts to take effect. It can be seen that all the factors which have been discussed in this chapter (as well as exercise, which is yet to be debated) have an effect upon a person's energy expenditure. All these factors must therefore be considered when contemplating how much to eat.

The importance of a regular weight check cannot be overemphasised for the aspiring sportsperson. It is the simplest method, available to us all, of monitoring the delicate energy balance.

3

Specific Requirements for Sport

In the preceding chapter it was illustrated that energy expenditure could be related directly to the level of physical work involved. In basic terms sport is not different. The energy expended in sport is the same as the energy involved in performing work and the basic calculations involved are also the same. For example, it is possible to calculate the amount of physical work done in the course of a 100m sprint by measuring the displacement of the centre of gravity and multiplying it by the number of strides taken during the course of the sprint. In much the same way as in the previous chapter regarding chores and occupational work, so researchers have made calculations for most of the sporting activities likely to be considered. The range varies from archery to wrestling and those activities omitted from the list can be assimilated by combining together certain other activities; for example, throwing and running combined might approximate the energy and skill of a Rugby back.

When looking at the effect that exercise has upon energy expenditure it becomes immediately apparent that the situation varies considerably with the degree of 'involvement'. The involvement factor can vary in players, events or in the same player from match to match. The level at which the game is played could also, theoretically, influence the degree of energy expenditure. While it is possible to use average levels when making such calculations, the keen statistician will make an accurate game analysis of a particular sportsperson, logging each time a specific movement is performed, making a note of the intensity of the effort so that a more accurate picture can be constructed. The game analysis, mainly used for establishing specific training programmes, is fast becoming a tool of the trade for the highly motivated coach or performer.

While the game or competition is the end-product of the sportsperson's efforts, most people who aspire to high levels of performance actually put more time and effort into their training. For example, it is not unusual for a top Wimbledon tennis player to practise for several hours

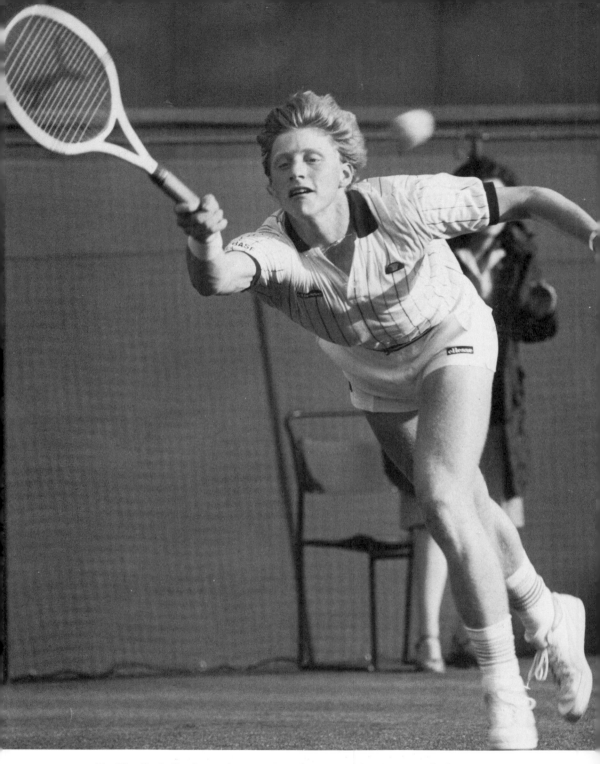

Fig 13 Boris Becker, who practises for several hours, even before a Wimbledon final.

almost immediately before going on to the centre court for the final. Certainly most world-class athletes train for several hours each day, when their competition might only last seconds. It is my firm belief that success in sport is in direct proportion to the amount of quality training (from which the sportsperson is able to recover quickly) that the athlete completes. Training must be regarded as a physiological investment account – the more you put in the more you can take out at a future date. Using the same analogy, the interest rates are higher when the investment is made under the direction of a well-qualified coach – the analagous financial adviser.

The training factors that influence energy expenditure are:

> the duration or period of effort
> the frequency or extent of effort
> the intensity or volume of effort

These are the three main variables in any training programme, but particularly so for those using an intermittent work principle. This principle is applied in a type of training in which periods of effort are interspersed with periods of recovery. In terms of energy consumption the greatest drain on the system is usually caused by the intensity of the effort. If the intensity is high, energy is used at a high rate and the stores are rapidly depleted. This situation will automatically force longer periods for recovery, less frequent repetitions and a considerably reduced duration of effort. With reference to the previous chapter, the energy system most likely to be used in such a situation is the anaerobic, in which waste products are built up and which have an inhibiting effect upon continuous exercise. For example, during a 100m (110yd) sprint, energy is being used at the rate of 51kcal per minute for the norm body-weight of 68kg (150lb), whereas running at a rate of one mile (1,500m) every five minutes requires something less than half of this value.

However, because there are so many variables in training sessions, it is quite likely that both the sprinter and the distance runner will have expended the same amount of energy at the end of their training. In the case of the sprinter, the intensity of effort limits the duration, and in the case of the distance runner the lower level of intensity permits a much longer period of effort. For example:

> 3 mins sprinting at 51kcal/min   =   153kcal
> 6 mins distance running at 25 kcal/min =   150kcal

Skill can also have a very considerable effect upon energy consumption. One frequently hears that the skilled performer 'makes it look easy'. Of course there is the naturally gifted player who has the ability to conserve energy. Likewise, there is the player who through practice has perfected his or her skill. In both situations such factors as anticipation, timing, balance, fluidity and relaxation enable the muscles to work without the added resistance of an opposing muscle group. Indeed, all unnecessary movements are eliminated and the muscles are allowed to work efficiently, so reducing the level of energy consumption. Consider a game such as tennis in which a match can last several hours. The practised skills of anticipation, balance and timing are all vital if high-level effort is to continue. Frequently, in very close, hard-fought contests, the result is determined by an endurance factor; either the player who has conserved energy during the early stages of the game or the player who, through training, has been able to build up greater reserves of energy will emerge the victor.

The latter statement suggests that energy reserves can be influenced by training, a statement no longer supported merely by supposition, but by proven physiological research. Training certainly increases an individual's glycogen reserves so that more energy-releasing substances are available. Glycogen reserves can also be influenced by diet, as in the case of carbohydrate loading (a system which will be discussed in Chapter 13). The basic physiological principle involved is that the body always adapts to stress (in this case the stress of glycogen depletion) by overcompensating and making more reserves available for future occasions.

However, the effects of training are not limited to energy reserves alone. High levels of physical activity produce waste products which accumulate and restrict levels of exercise, ultimately causing it to cease. The body has reserves which can counteract this acid situation, so permitting a higher level, or an extended period, of exercise. This reserve of alkaline materials, known as blood buffers, can be improved by as much as twelve per cent through selective training methods. Training at the correct level also familiarises the sportsperson to the stress of fatigue – building up a certain resistance to the situation. The human body is a magnificent machine; it has the capacity to turn some of our waste products into energy-giving substances. This system is further enhanced by training and, to a certain extent, by diet.

To summarise, training has the collective effect of improving an individual's endurance capacity by naturally increasing the reserves of energy, by excreting and neutralising acids, by facilitating a degree of reconstitution of waste products into energy-releasing substances and by familiarising the athlete with fatigue so that the body can be driven on when all else is telling it to stop. Roger Bannister, the first ever four-minute miler, might well have been right when he said 'Perhaps the razor's edge for victory is set rather by the psychological than the physiological.'

Following this preliminary discussion, introducing both the participation in sport and training for sport, it is obvious that the energy requirements for fuelling this involvement is considerably influenced both by the nature of a specific sport and by the type of training regime imposed upon the individual by the specific nature of that sport. For example, there is a considerable difference between the rather sedentary sport of bowls and the energy-demanding sport of Rugby football. However,

Activity	kcal/min
archery	5.2
badminton (competition)	10.0
basketball	6.0–9.0
boxing (amateur)	10.0–15.0
callisthenics	5.0
cycling (8–24kph (5–15mph))	5.0–12.0
football (association)	9.0
hurdling	21.3
judo or karate	13.0
jumping	7.0
rowing (competition)	15.0
running (400m/min (440yd)/min)	92.0
running (1 mile (1,600m) in 5min)	25.0
skating (competition)	10.0
sprinting (100m (110yd))	51.0
squash	10.0
swimming (60m/min (66yd)/min)	29.2
swimming (70m/min (77yd)/min)	35.1
throwing	12.6
walking (8kph (5mph))	11.3
wrestling	14.4

Fig 14   This table is taken from W. Paish, Diet in Sport, and is based on work done by Yakovlev in the Soviet Union and Sharkey of the USA. The table lists a number of sports and gives the energy expenditure, in kilocalories per minute, for each sport. It assumes a body-weight of 68kg (150lb); for every 7kg (15lb) above this figure, ten per cent should be added to the figure in the second column. Similarly for every 7kg (15lb) below 68kg (150lb), ten per cent should be subtracted.

other than activities such as marathon running, most sports are of an intermittent nature whereby periods of very high activity are interspersed with periods of relative inactivity. A classic example of this is the fast bowler in cricket, who is extremely active for one over, but is then permitted a period of greatly reduced activity while the bowler from the other end attempts to bowl out the batsman.

Researchers have compiled energy tables for most sports which allow for the intermittent nature of play and so represent the average player in the average game. Nevertheless an individual game analysis will always provide more accurate information, should it be required. I would recommend the game-analysis approach for any top-class sportsperson who wishes to have his or her body in perfect condition.

The list in Fig 14 is by no means complete. Chapters 8–12 are devoted to the calculation of energy requirements for specific sports and discuss the requirements for typical individuals involved in those sports.

4
Specific Requirements for Women

Although in the western world we live in a culture of almost total emancipation, with women holding down key posts in most walks of life, sport has only paid lip service to the special needs of women in respect of their sporting endeavours. It has to be accepted that women can never be the equal of men in any sport influenced by strength and endurance. Their physiological structure militates against such equality. However, in sports where the determining factor is skill, equality can exist. In power- and endurance-based sports, the nearest the female approaches the male is in long-distance swimming, where women's higher levels of fat aid flotation and reduce the difference in performance to as little as ten per cent.

The physiological structure of the woman was created to bear children. Thus it imposes both anatomical and physiological limitations on them in sport which are not experienced by men. Up to the early stages of puberty the performance of boys and girls can be considered equal. This equality is clearly the case in track and field athletics; both in sprinting and middle-distance running, girls frequently emerge as victors. However, after puberty, the strength and endurance factors, naturally higher in men, start to take over and make the difference of which we are all aware.

Because of their different physiological make-up, women must regard their needs, so far as nutrition is concerned, as different from those of men, especially if they are keen to compete in peak condition. In a normal society, the average woman eats an almost identical diet to the average man. However, I hope that most sections of this book have emphasised that people involved in sport, especially at high levels, cannot be considered as average and that they present quite a different problem regarding their nutrition.

In terms of basic nutrients, in order to provide energy to fuel muscular effort, there is no significant difference between men and women.

47

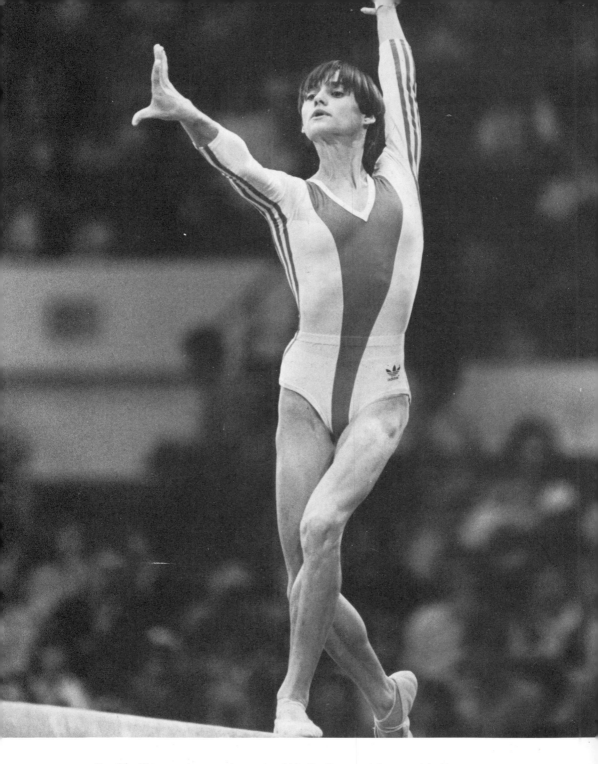

Fig 15 The near-anorexic state of Nadia Comaneci, a world-class
gymnast. Anorexia was later diagnosed.

Hence, those differences which do exist must be attributed to the effect of the female hormones, oestrogen and progesterone and to the effects which these have upon the body. Only very recently have gynaecologists started to take an interest in sport, to realise that sport is affected by women's cyclical changes and that sport itself affects these changes. It must also be understood that any treatment designed to reduce irregularities in the cycle will affect performance in sport. A pioneer in this area was Andrew Mathews, a consultant gynaecologist at the West Middlesex Hospital, who was invited by Marea Hartman, the British team manager at the 1968 Olympic games, to help in the preparations of the British team. These two people, working together, brought a new dimension to sport for women in the United Kingdom.

The onset of menstruation starts at about 11–13 years of age. At this stage the cycle is irregular and ovulation seldom exists, although the amount of blood lost can be in the region of 50–150ml (1.8–5.3 fl.oz.) This therefore, must be taken into account when considering nutritional needs. Sport can influence the onset of menstruation, usually delaying it by several years, especially when the training levels are high. There are no harmful side-effects caused by this delay, but the diet of girls at this stage needs to be planned carefully to restrict the associated weight gains and to guard against anaemia.

In the adult woman changes are more significant. The fourteen days prior to ovulation are influenced by oestrogen. The mood this creates is cheerful and buoyant and is ideal for injecting heavy training loads. After ovulation, gestagens become more evident and the mood frequently changes to produce the symptoms known as pre-menstrual tension (PMT). Research indicates that at least eighty per cent of women suffer from PMT with over forty per cent experiencing quite unpleasant side-effects, which include: irritability; depression; breast pains; bloated sensations due to fluid retention; headaches; clumsiness; swollen ankles; reduced libido; constipation; hot flushes; back ache; nausea; lethargy; and a craving for something like chocolate, which can have an effect upon the energy balance, as well as making the side-effects of PMT more pronounced.

Other than the time immediately before ovulation, there are marked cyclical changes which can influence performance in sport. Research statistics indicate that prior to menstruation lung function is at a maximum, as is pulse rate, whereas muscular co-ordination is at its lowest. There is also an increased susceptibility to infections, accidents and injuries. Diet can influence the PMT syndrome and a well-planned diet, at this stage of the menstrual cycle, can bring about quite marked transformations. This is essential for those women who wish to compete in sport at a high level.

PMT can be exacerbated by the effects of fatty acids upon prostaglandin E_1 – which normally has a regulating effect upon oestrogen and progesterone during the important phase of the cycle. Several research articles list the benefits of a substance called evening primrose oil and of the stabilising effect which zinc has upon the system. Hence supplementation of the diet with these two elements could help those who suffer badly. However, the symptoms seem to be more affected by what should not be done during this phase rather than by what should be done. Several researchers have found that by avoiding tea and coffee in particular, the serious nature of the symptoms is considerably reduced. For those addicted to the beverages, herbal and fruit teas make excellent substitutes and do not promote any of the disturbing side-effects of the former. Other foods which rate highly on the list of things to be avoided are chocolate, sugar, salt and dairy products. Smoking also has an adverse effect upon the system, although many women become reliant upon the effect of the drug to ease any pain.

Research into the side-effects of the contraceptive pill varies according to the source. There is roughly an equal split between those who suggest that the pill amplifies the condition and those who suggest that the condition is made less painful by taking the pill. While research continues, it would appear that individuals react differently.

Although the average woman during the pre-menstrual phase may regard exercise as a little like 'rubbing salt into the wound', the fact remains that exercise is beneficial in reducing the discomfort of PMT, probably due to the effect which exercise has upon the endocrine system and hence the sex hormones. Indeed, the modern woman athlete now trains through this phase and has learned to cope with the effects of the cyclic changes. Participants in a number of sports, of which track and field athletics is one, have attempted to regulate the monthly cycle leading up to major competitions by the extended use of the contraceptive pill. This is done to avoid competitions coinciding with the PMT phase. However, for many, the unpleasant side-effects associated with the casual use of the pill far outweigh any of the beneficial effects which might be experienced.

Dr Judy Graham, in her book *Evening Primrose Oil*, a text devoted to the therapeutic use of this substance, explains in detail how the essential fatty acid, linoleic acid, aids the production of prostaglandins and how in turn these are aided by the presence of vitamins B and E and by zinc and magnesium. However, of equal significance is how those beneficial effects are blocked by the presence of too much saturated fat; cholesterol; alcohol; low blood-sugar level and the resultant effect upon the sugar-effective hormones; by the effect of the stress-related hormones, adrenaline, nor-adrenaline and cortisol; by ageing; by zinc deficiency; and by viral infections. Dr Graham also illustrates how evening primrose oil can help in the final metabolic changes of linoleic acid towards the production of prostaglandin E_1 and again how the water-soluble vitamins can help in this reaction.

From a personal viewpoint, from the experience I have had working with a large number of excellent women athletes, I have found that heavy training loads, in particular with distance runners, has reduced body-fat levels to the extent where this has caused a disruption of the monthly cycle, but without any obvious ill-effects. I have also come across cases in which PMT has sadly affected both training and competition results; one athlete could even induce a very heavy period only minutes before a major competition, due to the stressful nature of top-level competitive sport.

Apart from the relief which the pill might give to PMT sufferers, some sportswomen will be taking the pill for contraceptive reasons or to regulate both the intensity and duration of blood-flow. These situations will have an effect upon the diet. It is well established that taking the pill has an adverse effect upon the body in that it depletes the level of the water-soluble vitamins and also reduces the availability of magnesium and zinc, while at the same time increasing the level of copper.

Magnesium is needed for energy production and for protein synthesis. The woman athlete will require a daily amount of about 300µg. While it is found in sufficient amounts in milk, nuts and seeds, it must be accepted that cooking has an adverse effect upon its availability. Zinc is certainly the most important mineral that can have an effect upon PMT. It is required for the correct function of all of our vital organs and has an enzymic effect upon the utilisation of most vitamins. Zinc levels are lowest during the pre-menstrual syndrome and therefore may require supplementation or an increase in the amount of seafood in the daily diet.

Vitamin B_6 has been found to play an important role in the treatment of PMT. It, too, has a co-enzymic effect upon the conversion of fatty acids. Research has established that the contraceptive pill considerably reduces the level of vitamin B_6 and so in order to assure the availability of about 150mg per day some form of supplementation may be necessary. The fact that the contraceptive pill decreases the availability of vitamin C can have quite disastrous effects upon performance standards. Its association with the absorption of iron is well illustrated elsewhere in this text and does not require further amplification. So too is its effect upon fighting viral infections such as the common cold. However, its effects upon reducing fluid retention, particularly in the lower limbs, is not well documented. Therefore I would recommend that those women who take the contra-ceptive pill should supplement vitamin C by as much as 3g per day. Unfortunately eating citrus fruit is unlikely to produce such levels of this vitamin and so supplementation is the only obvious solution.

Without doubt, sports nutritionists, coaches and the like must be aware of women's needs and take into account the cyclic changes when planning diets and training. While training programmes can be similar to men's the cyclic changes must force a careful examination of the diet. To summarise, I would certainly recommend that ambitious sportswomen supplement their diets with:

> evening primrose oil (up to 3g per day)
> vitamin C (up to 3g per day)
> vitamin B_6 (up to 150mg per day, with
> some added total vitamin B complex)
> vitamin E (up to 300mg per day)
> and zinc (up to 10mg per day)

Of course, most of these can be found in a general mineral/vitamin complex, all in one capsule, which companies have made specifically for women – so avoiding taking a large number of different pills for each vitamin or mineral. I appreciate that such a recommendation might seem to be a harsh criticism of one's normal diet, but I am convinced that any sacrifice will be amply rewarded by enhanced performances in sport.

5

Food and Sport

This chapter considers food, its basic constituents and its importance with specific reference to sport, as well as the examination of how certain nutrients might contribute towards an enhanced performance.

Carbohydrates

About sixty or seventy per cent of a sportsperson's diet should come in the form of carbohydrates. Those involved in 'ultra-endurance' events might even need to go beyond seventy per cent for short periods of time, especially following exhaustive training.

During rest it is generally accepted that the metabolic requirements are met by using a combination of the three basic nutrients: carbohydrates; fats; and proteins – which should, respectively, form 42, 41 and 17 per cent of the body's energy requirements. However, during exercise these proportions can change dramatically when affected by the intensity (severity) and the extent (volume) of the exercise. When the intensity of exercise is more than sixty-five per cent of $\dot{V}O_{2max}$ (see Glossary) and of short duration (less than an hour), carbohydrates are the major source of energy. During prolonged bouts of exercise at the same intensity, fats become the prime source of energy. Under normal circumstances protein is not an important source of energy, although recent research suggests that at very intense levels of exercise proteins make a significant contribution to energy supplies, mainly because there is insufficient oxygen to metabolise fats.

As the body can store carbohydrates in the form of glycogen (to the order of about 2,500kcal), it is without doubt the body's primary source of energy. Because glycogen is the basic fuel for exercise and is used even for the production of energy from protein, carbohydrates tend to have a rationing effect upon the use of protein as an energy provider. Moreover, they also serve as a primer for the use of fatty acids. It is generally accepted that carbohydrates form no useful function in the

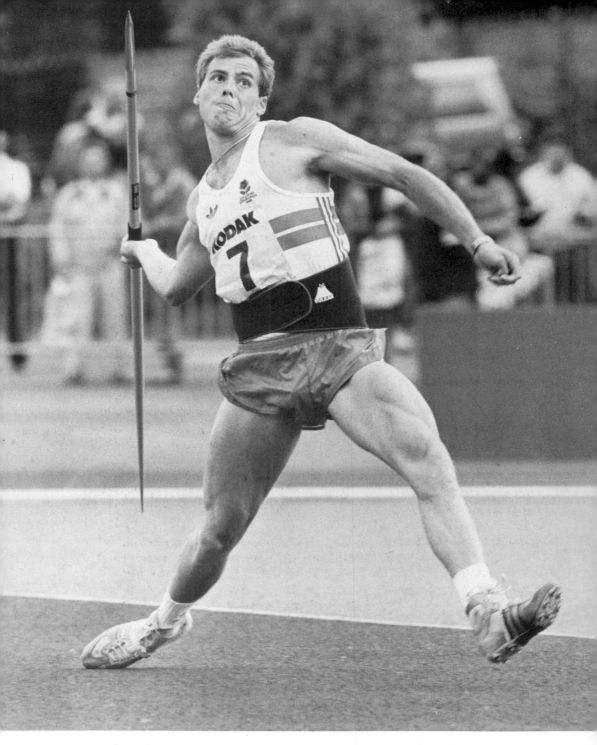

Fig 16   Mick Hill, who through careful training and eating has
produced a physique capable of matching the best throwers in the
world.

body other than as a primary source of energy. In many respects this is true, since they do not bind any vitamins and they do not contribute to a hormone pool. Nevertheless, a healthy life cannot be led without them since the nervous system can only function efficiently on energy derived from carbohydrates. Moreover, they are essential for sport so they must contribute to well over half of the sportsperson's diet.

As mentioned earlier, carbohydrates exist in two forms – starches and sugars. It is now well established that the sportsperson requires most of the necessary carbohydrates in the form of complex starches. Russian research dating back to 1961, by Yakovlev, suggested that people involved in high-level sport need at least sixty-four per cent of their carbohydrate intake in the form of starch and only thirty-six per cent in the form of sugars. More recent research puts the level at eighty per cent for the complex starches. There is also some evidence to indicate that sugars act as an irritant to the digestive, endocrine and nervous systems. Its associated effect on the endocrine system is well documented, in particular the effect of a large ingestion of sugar upon the sugar-responsive hormones. This came to light when sportspeople started to use glucose drinks and tablets in the belief that they might increase blood-sugar levels, only to find that the reverse was the case (because of the homoeostatic response of insulin).

A number of researchers have found that by increasing the intake of carbohydrates the muscle glycogen levels are considerably increased. Of particular relevence is the work done by Sharman et al. in 1984. His team of researchers found that while doubling the intake of carbohydrates had little effect upon pre-exercise levels of muscle glycogen, the effect upon a 24-hour post-exercise level is dramatic, an increase in the region of forty per cent. This indicates that the carbohydrates are used to restock energy supplies following exercise. It is also well established that the stores of muscle glycogen are best replaced by an ingestion of carbohydrates as quickly as possible after exercise and certainly within forty-five minutes of depletion; otherwise it can take over forty-eight hours to return the reserves to normal. Herein lies a problem for most sportspeople and certainly for the majority of top-class athletes. Very strenuous activity has an inhibiting effect upon appetite and most sportspeople are unlikely to want to eat anything substantial for several hours after exercise and certainly not during the recommended time of forty-five minutes. Also, most good-class sportspeople will have exercised again before the upper limit for repletion of forty-eight hours has been reached. Indeed many athletes would have trained at least twice within this period of time. This means that subsequent training sessions commence with low glycogen reserves and because this can be cumulative complete fatigue may result. This situation presents the sportsperson with two possible solutions.

The first is to attempt to replenish the reserves as quickly as possible. Very few foods are palatable soon after vigorous exercise, but apples and grapes, which contain the right ingredients to start the replenishment cycle, are more acceptable than most. From a purely practical point of view I have found that apples travel better in the training bag and they are also ideal so far as cost is concerned. So the old saying 'an apple a day' might have a new meaning in sport. Certainly, unlike glucose drinks, there is little fear of the insulin response being activated. Following research by Andrew Bosch, of the University of Cape Town medical school, a number of people involved in very high-level endurance events have started to experiment with carbohydrate polymer drinks. Research indicates that these specially prepared drinks, which are now on the market, are significantly more beneficial than glucose and sucrose drinks. The drinks are marketed under the name of F.R.N. squeezy and are offered in a variety of flavours.

The second avenue open for sportspeople to make sure that muscle glycogen levels and liver glycogen reserves are replenished is to take periods of rest between exhaustive training sessions. Indeed I favour a cycle of training which comprises one day hard, two days very hard and one day of complete rest in a four-day training programme. Carbohydrates are easily obtained in the diet as most of our common foods are high in this nutrient. For example bread and cereals are between fifty and seventy per cent carbohydrate and potatoes fifteen per cent. The charts listed in Appendix 1 will also serve as a guide for other foods rich in this nutrient. It is unlikely that any diet, excluding those affected by drought, will be deficient in carbohydrate.

So far, there has been no discussion of carbohydrate loading, first advanced by Saltin in the 1960s. The theory supporting carbohydrate loading is very sound, but does not always work out in practice. This diet will be discussed more fully in the final chapter.

To summarise – it should be obvious to the reader that carbohydrates have a very profound effect upon many aspects of sports nutrition and they must be regarded as the foundation of energy building.

Fats

While most texts on nutrition highlight only the possible ill-effects of too much dietary fat, it must be emphasised that they are essential for life and represent a massive potential store of energy which most active sports-people will need to tap. The criticisms of high-fat diets are all associated with obesity and the net results of overburdening the body with excess weight. There is also the association of cholesterol and fats with heart disease. However, it is fairly certain that fats alone will not cause adverse heart conditions; they are rather just one of a number of contributory factors.

Many women in sport try to train on an almost fat-free diet, the result often being anorexia and all of the resultant side-effects of this illness. Obviously, such a diet should be avoided.

Fats are stored in white adipose tissue cells and in skeletal muscle. The average man has a fat store which represents about fifteen per cent of his body-weight, while the average woman has a store of about twenty per cent. It is certain that those involved in heavy training loads will be well below these average figures. Many middle- and long-distance runners frequently reduce their fat levels to as little as five per cent for men and ten per cent for women. It is very important to note here that there is a significant gender difference; when a woman's body-fat content drops below about twelve per cent amenorrhoea is induced.

Most of the fat stored is available as a fuel to provide energy for exercise. The more fat that is used, the less is the body's reliance upon glycogen. Glycogen must be stored in a water-based solution whereas fats are anhydrous and so offer a greater energy:weight ratio. Another significant fact is that during oxidation 1g of fat yields 9.3kcal whereas 1g of carbohydrate yields 4kcal. Also, when training for endurance events one of the body's natural feedback loops stimulates the body to oxidise fat in order to fuel the working muscles. The resultant effect is that the trained endurance athlete can call upon fat reserves before depleting those of glycogen.

The potential energy in fats is circulated to the skeletal muscles in the form of fatty acids. These fatty acids are not used for energy but can be used to top up the store of glycogen in the liver or be converted back to fat again and stored as adipose tissue. The metabolism of fats is an aerobic process and it can produce a potential store of energy larger than that provided by the aerobic metabolism of glycogen.

Skeletal muscles are composed of three types of muscle fibres, known as fast, medium and slow glycolytic. The different fibres use glycogen at different rates. During slower, sustained work the slow fibres provide most of the input and these fibres will fatigue first at this level of exercise. It is this group of fibres that has the greater capacity to use fats as an energy source. Research has shown that when exercising at a rate of seventy to seventy-five per cent of $\dot{V}O_{2max}$, carbohydrates are the main source of energy during the first hour and during subsequent periods of effort the change is towards a fat dominance. At exercise levels in excess of seventy-five per cent of $\dot{V}O_{2max}$ all three fibres must be used and energy is provided by the stores of ATP and PC and as such the period of exercise is considerably reduced.

The above discussion has been used to demonstrate that fats make a very valuable contribution to the athlete's energy store, and in many cases provide over twenty per cent of the total available. However, fats also contribute to the efficiency of the sportsperson in a number of other ways. They bind the fat-soluble vitamins A, D, E and K (*see* Fig 12 on page 39). Fats also contribute to the enzyme pool and the steroid group in particular fit into the chain of fats. Following the disqualification of the 1988 Olympic 100m 'champion' Ben Johnson for taking anabolic steroids even greater attention has been focused upon drug abuse in sport. This is discussed in Chapter 6 on ergogenic aids. Here it is sufficient to say that many aspects of homoeostasis, and in particular that related to exercise, is controlled by steroids which in turn relate to our dietary fats.

Also included in the fat chain is a phospholipid known as lecithin, which many people in sport take as a supplement. The supporting principle of this supplementation is based on the fact that lecithin surrounds nervous tissue – so acting as an insulator for the network. As neuromuscular impulses are electro-chemical by nature, it would follow that a well-insulated fibre might transmit a more efficient response.

In conclusion, fats are essential for prolonged health. They represent a massive potential store of energy for people involved in sport, they bind vitamins and promote homoeostasis through the action of hormones. However, they should not be taken in excess, particularly for those who lead a sedentary lifestyle as excessive fat intake has a very close relationship with the incidence of coronary heart disease. It is my opinion that this is unlikely to be the case with the very active sportsperson who uses in excess of 3,000kcal per day.

Protein

In recent years the subject of protein has become almost as emotive for people involved in sport as that of vitamins. Those who believe that the active body requires more protein will not be moved from their desire to supplement this nutrient. Indeed the vogue term in sports nutrition at the moment is 'free-form amino acids'. Very recent research, albeit originally

Amino acid	Possible function
lysine*	aids transportation of fatty acids to mitochondria, works in conjunction with vitamin C as a virus fighter
methionine*	a detoxicant, aids certain enzyme activity
phenylalanine*	aids the production and conversion of other amino acids
tryptophan*	essential for the correct functioning of nervous tissue, exercises a control over the metabolism
threonine*	has an effect, through the nervous system, upon concentration and personality
valine*	helps the efficiency of skeletal muscle
histidine*	aids the growth of skeletal muscle, helps to promote a healthy nervous system
arginine*	has a marked effect upon testosterone levels, helps in energy production through glycolysis, promotes growth through hormone activity
leucine*	helps as a detoxicant during anaerobic work
proline	helps in tissue rebuilding in conjunction with vitamin C
taurine	has an effect associated with the secretion of the female hormones (oestrogen and progesterone)
carnitine	helps the metabolism of fats for energy, works in conjunction with vitamin C
tyrosine	promotes a healthy nervous system
glutamine glutamic acid	both act as detoxicants
glycine	a detoxicant, helps in the balance of nitrogen
ornithine	enhances the performance of the liver, stimulates growth hormone activity

Fig 17   Amino acids and their possible functions. This list is by no means comprehensive; only those amino acids which have a recognised effect particularly useful to the sportsperson are given. Careful reading of the functions of arginine and ornithine will explain why these two amino acids are especially popular with sportspeople. Those amino acids essential to life are marked with an asterisk. Isoleucine (not mentioned in the list) is also in this latter category.

59

intended to make the sick well, has established that certain amino acids (*see* Fig 17) could have a most beneficial effect upon the physiological structure of the sportsperson. The market potential for individual amino acids has probably been stimulated by the increasingly strict application of the rules banning the use of performance-enhancing drugs and the more elaborate testing procedures used to detect their presence. There are indications that certain amino acids, through their effect upon hormones (in particular those affecting growth; the anabolic and andro-genic groups) might be a legal method of enhancing performance.

Controversy always exists, particularly in the area of sporting en-deavour, as to how much protein is actually needed by the body. Most nations in the world accept the general recommendation of 1g per kg (0.035oz per 2.2lb) of body-weight per day. However, those who re-search the situation in sport, and there are many such people producing a wealth of material, recommend 2g per kg (0.07oz per 2.2lb) per day for the active sportsperson. This is certainly very sound advice when one considers protein in terms of energy alone, since the average person involved in sport requires about twice as much energy as the more sedentary person.

If the body does not get sufficient protein during food ingestion, the cell-rebuilding process cannot take place and certain vital tissues will waste away. There is also the very well established fact that protein has a profound effect upon essential enzymes, hormones and blood-cell pro-duction. Conversely, if too much protein is ingested, the excess has to be used for energy which produces a toxic by-product, caused by the removal of the nitrogen part of the molecule, so producing a substance known as urea.

Very recent research is now highlighting the fact that changes in muscle protein during and following exercise is difficult to explain, raising the possibility that coaches could be forced to change their training techniques in order to bring about a different adaptive response. Certainly, this is a very complicated field and much research waits to be carried out.

Vitamins

Most of what has been written so far has been concerning the provision of energy from the three basic nutrients. As these nutrients are contained in most common foods it is unlikely that anyone involved in sport will be deficient in these nutrients to the extent that they cannot meet their energy demands. As discussed earlier, it is fairly easy to decide how much energy is required and in what proportions the basic nutrients make their contribution. The same cannot be said about vitamins. The reason is that their precise action is still not fully understood. They are only required in very small amounts and their primary source is often not easy to recognise. With this level of uncertainty, the field has become cluttered with myths and legends, fallacies, old wives' tales and the occasional fact, so creating a situation which lends itself to commercial exploitation.

The various vitamins together with the common sources are listed in Fig 18. Mention is also made as to their general effect upon the body and how they serve as catalysts, making the chemical processes involved in nutrition more effective.

From regular contact with sportsmen and women of the highest level, two points regarding athletes' diets have become clear to me. The first is that most athletes will not be deficient in energy-giving foods, although an exception to this might be some international-class women distance runners. The second point is that as most athletes eat a fairly narrow variety of food the chances are that they will be deficient in vitamins, so making it unlikely that any of them can work at peak efficiency. To correct this situation the sportsperson *must* eat a good selection of fresh fruit and vegetables and then supplement this diet where necessary. While I am a keen supporter of vitamin therapy it must not be used indiscriminately; supplements cannot take the place of good, natural food.

While there is much documentary evidence to identify the action and sources of the various vitamins, there is very little on how, when and in what quantities vitamins are really required. Shortly before the second period of Finnish dominance of middle-distance running in the 1970s (when New Zealand was the leading nation at these events) researchers compared the lifestyles of the Finnish athletes and the New Zealand stars. A major identifiable difference was one of nutrition association with the greater availability of green vegetables in New Zealand. Soon after the Finns placed greater emphasis on nutrition, the achievements of their athletes improved.

Figs 19 to 21 provide recommended intakes for differing vitamins. Fig 19 lists these recommendations for athletes during different stages of their training and shows the approved figures as compiled by a Russian researcher from the Department of Physical Culture in Moscow in 1961, N. N. Yakovlev. (*See* Chapter 9.) These values are designed for athletes of international standard. Fig 20 is based on research carried out with top Finnish middle-distance runners in the 1970s, when they were the best in the world. Fig 21 gives the recommended values as used in the United Kingdom.

Vitamin	Action	Source
A	has an effect upon vision, healthy skin, teeth, epithelial tissue (respiratory tract and digestive tract)	eggs, milk, liver, carrots
B_1 (thyamine)	aids release of energy from carbohydrates, promotes healthy nervous tissue	yeast, nuts, bran, wheat-germ; depleted by contraceptive pill
B_2 (riboflavin)	aids the metabolism of basic nutrients	yeast, fish, green vegetables, kidney, liver, nuts
B_6 (pyridoxine)	helps in the assimilation of fats and carbohydrates, promotes the growth of red blood cells, needed for correct function of vitamin B_{12}	yeast, nuts, egg yolk, bananas
B_{12}	helps production of red blood cells, has a profound effect upon all cellular activity, especially muscle cells	liver, cheese, eggs, yeast, bananas
B_{15} (pangamic acid)	helps production of glycogen, minimises lactic acid production, helps metabolise fats for energy	yeast, fish
biotin	helps metabolism of fats and proteins	yeast, soya, kidney, bananas
choline	helps efficiency of cardiovascular system	yeast, liver, green vegetables, wheat-germ
folic acid	aids B_{12} and red cell production, keeps liver efficient	yeast, kidney, green vegetables, mushrooms
inositol	helps transport and metabolism of fats	yeast, milk, citrus fruit, nuts
iodine	helps production of ATP	yeast, nuts
nicotinic acid	aids digestion and release of energy from fats and carbohydrates	yeast, nuts, green vegetables, rice
pantothenic acid	wide spectrum effect, aids energy release from fats and carbohydrates	yeast, egg yolk, green vegetables
vitamin C	promotes general health of all tissues, fights viruses and aids absorption of iron	citrus fruit, green vegetables

Vitamin	Action	Source
vitamin D (calciferol)	aids growth and health of bones, helps absorption of calcium	sunlight, fish, butter, milk
vitamin E	helps oxygen uptake, helps injury-healing rate and red blood-cell formation, increases testosterone levels, helps form prostaglandins, aids use of vitamin A	nuts, wheat, eggs, green vegetables
vitamin K	helps conversion of amino acids, aids blood clotting	green vegetables

Fig 18   Vitamins, their likely effects upon the body and their main sources.

It is interesting to note (in Fig 21) that in terms of sport 3,600kcal is not really very active. Indeed if this is compared with either Fig 19 or 20, based on the Russian and Finnish work, it can be seen that these represent twice as much as the UK recommendations. This can perhaps be explained by the fact that the UK recommendations assume an energy expenditure of roughly half the other tables.

It is always interesting to talk to sportspeople about their eating habits and, in particular, what they supplement. It is particularly interesting to compare people from different nations, especially those from the USA. Here for example, most athletes supplement with vitamins, while only about ten per cent of the British team do so. However, there is now some evidence that this is changing and that British sportspeople are now looking more towards some vitamin supplementation. There is also a vast difference between sports; for example, body-builders will examine their diet in the same detail as their training schedule. On the other hand the athlete and major games player pays little more than lip service to the supporting role of nutrition. The reason for this situation could be ignorance, lack of specific education, a belief that one's diet is already correct and that it will provide all the nutrients that are required. The problem now, for the average sportsperson, is that it is difficult to distinguish healthy eating from the health-food market – and much of what is written about food and supplementation comes from people with a vested interest. However, there is much valid research published to support what is said in this advertising material and indeed all advertising is subject to the strictest medical supervision in order to protect the public from exploitation. Personally, I am an avid supporter of supplementation, but only after a careful examination of the existing diet.

Training period	Explosive events A B₁ B₂ B₃ C E (mg)						Endurance events A B₁ B₂ B₃ C E (mg)					
active recovery	2.0	2.5	2.0	20	75	3.0	2.0	3.0	2.0	20	100	3.0
principal training	3.0	5.0	2.5	20	150	3.0	3.0	1.0	5.0	25	250	6.0
competition period	2.0	1.0	5.0	20	150	3.0	2.0	1.5	5.0	25	300	6.0

Fig 19   The recommended vitamin intake for athletes during different phases of training.

vitamin	A	B₁	B₂	B₃	C	E
intake (mg)	3.3	2.5–5.0	2.6–5.0	20	100–250	30–60

Fig 20   The recommended vitamin intake for top-class distance runners, as used by Finnish athletes during the early 1970s.

Occupation	Energy requirement (kcal)	B₁ (mg)	B₂	B₃	C	A (μg)	D
sedentary	2,700	1.1	1.7	18	30	0.75	2.5
moderately active	3,000	1.2	1.7	18	30	0.75	2.5
very active	3,600	1.4	1.8	18	30	0.75	2.5

Fig 21   The recommended vitamin intake for people leading sedentary or more active lives (figures prepared for use in the United Kingdom).

Fig 18 on pages 62 and 63 gives a general picture of the importance of vitamins; this section aims to be more specific and to relate the role of vitamins directly to sport.

Vitamin A

Lack of vitamin A can produce an effect similar to night-blindness, a situation in which vision is impaired in diminishing and artificial light. As many competitions, such as floodlit games, now take place under such conditions, sportspeople should ensure that they are not disadvantaged by a deficiency of this vitamin. Vitamin A also has a very positive effect upon growth, mainly through its action on protein metabolism. The two work together to produce the anabolic (building up) effect, a situation which many sportspeople are keen to achieve. Vitamin A is a favourite with body-builders because they are convinced of its value in muscle building. It is a fat-soluble vitamin and, if taken in excess, could have an effect upon the liver and become toxic. It is present in significant amounts in eggs and dairy products. Those who avoid these foods would need to look towards less productive sources such as carrots and green, leafy vegetables – or even supplementation.

Vitamin B Group

This is the group most likely to have a significant effect upon sports performance. While the group is numbered up to sixteen, most of them are identical in their chemical composition, although B_1, B_2, B_6 and B_{12} are significantly different. There is also a very close interaction between the members of the group to produce an orchestrated effect upon the body.

Quite a number of nations who have an admirable sporting record recommend vitamin B therapy to their international stars. B_1, B_2 and B_3 (niacin) have an effect upon carbohydrate metabolism and upon the production of energy, certainly at mitochondria level. B_{12} is more specifically associated with producing the ultimate form of energy – ATP. Personal observations and discussion with athletes at the major athletic championships in the period leading up to the 1988 Olympic games indicated that power-based sportpeople were using injections of B_{12} (cyanocobalamin) and ATP in an attempt to improve their anaerobic capacity. While most critics would suggest that its effect can only be as a placebo – and as a coach I would agree that this is a legitimate use, since it does not contravene the rules on doping – I find it very hard not to accept that its effect must be physiological and that some nations are more advanced in this field than others.

Vitamins B_6, B_{12} and folic acid have a recognised effect upon the body's capacity to produce red blood-cells and injections of these vitamins are frequently used in the treatment of anaemia (a disease which causes a reduced level of haemoglobin). This condition is very common in sport and considerably restricts efficiency especially as far as endurance is concerned.

The vitamin B group also has an effect upon the efficiency of the nervous system, and those who have low levels of this group of vitamins often display a lower capacity for concentration and reduced levels of co-ordination. Vitamin B_6 (pyridoxine) is also known to have an effect upon protein metabolism when protein is used as an energy source; this has been discussed earlier in this chapter.

Most of the B vitamins, with the exception of B_{12}, are found in cereal foods, especially those which have not been too refined. There are also significant levels in fish and meat (in particular liver). As the B group is water-soluble with an extremely short life-span they are unlikely to become toxic.

Vitamin C

This is probably the most familiar vitamin to the average person. It is recognised as the 'virus fighter' and many drink orange juice and eat oranges in an attempt to boost its availability. While in theory this is correct, it falls short in practice since very large doses of vitamin C are required to produce this desired effect and taking vitamin C in this form will have very little long-term effect. Vitamin C is a water-soluble vitamin. Stores are not built up in the body and so a daily intake is necessary to have any benefit.

Apart from the influence which vitamin C has upon helping a person's resistance to viral infections and its influence on the rate of healing, it also has a wider effect; it promotes the absorption of iron and as such helps to combat anaemia. Indeed vitamin C has such a total effect upon the whole area of metabolism that no sportsperson can afford to be without an adequate supply. Low levels certainly affect training performances which, in turn, detract from any ultimate goals.

Vitamin D

Calciferol has a dramatic effect upon calcium absorption and so controls the state of bone repair and the health of teeth. Those people involved in hard contact sports such as association and Rugby football are always in danger of bone damage. The repair of this damage is in part influenced by the presence of this vitamin.

Vitamin E

Many of the claims made of this vitamin, with specific reference to sport, cannot be substantiated. For example, just over a decade ago, researchers claimed that vitamin E had an effect upon the production of testosterone, the male sex hormone, although there has been little voiced on this subject recently. If this original work is authentic, it is easy to see how performance in sport could be altered by the anabolic and androgenic effect of testosterone.

Other research work in an entirely different field has indicated that vitamin E has an effect upon the injury healing rate, in particular that of superficial tissue. Most sportspeople involved in contact and combat sports receive injuries of this nature which, if slow to repair, can put a player out of the game for an extended period. A number of players, in particular the professionals, where income is related to performance, frequently turn out when in an injured state, so running the risk of further complications. This time away from the sport could in all probability be shortened through the natural processes of the body via a stimulation of vitamin E.

Vitamins A and C are unable to function correctly without the presence of vitamin E – yet another illustration of the interdependence of vitamins. Recent research, associated with the provision of energy from the fat sources, indicates that vitamin E also has an enzymic effect upon fat metabolism. All in all, people involved in sport cannot function at peak efficiency without an adequate supply of this fat-soluble vitamin.

Vitamin K

Vitamin K is the only remaining vitamin to complete the 'orchestra'; this has an effect upon the potential of the blood to clot. Sport is, of course, not without injury risk, so that both external and internal bleeding is accepted as just one of the hazards of the game. It would therefore appear obvious to ensure that levels of this vitamin are naturally high, which can be achieved by eating the correct foods, so allowing the process of healing to be undertaken efficiently. Vitamin K also aids the digestion of fats and, as stated earlier, the top sportsperson may, at some stage, derive in the region of fifty per cent of his or her total energy from this source.

Minerals

Minerals have two basic functions in the body, influencing the morphological structure and the metabolism of the body. Perhaps the most obvious mineral in the former category is calcium. It is easy to recognise that a considerable percentage of our body-weight is composed of this mineral. Calcium has an effect upon the formation, protection and repair of bone. It must be the concern of every active participant to make sure that this essential supporting and protective structure functions with peak efficiency. It is therefore essential to include a good supply of calcium in the diet.

Less obvious, but nevertheless of vital importance, is the action of iron. Its effect upon oxygen-carrying potential has been highlighted in other sections of this text. However, it is essential to appreciate fully its role so far as sport is concerned. The act of training has a profound effect upon red blood-cells. Once the heart rate is increased, the speed of circulation is also raised several times to take the nutrients to the active tissues and to transport waste products away. This speeding-up process causes the structure of the cells to deteriorate and produces the condition of anaemia. This illness is very common, in particular among women who take part in endurance events, although it must be stressed that the condition is not limited to women alone. However, it must be accepted that women can shed up to 70ml (2.5fl.oz.) of blood in a single menstrual period. If haemoglobin were not a constituent of blood the active body would need over 300l (530pt.) to transport sufficient oxygen to fuel strenuous activity. The human body would consequently have to be both massive and very strong in order to support such a volume of fluid and it would probably need to resemble a prehistoric monster! With haemoglobin, however, the body can cope with about 5l (8pt.) of blood, although on occasions it is forced around the body several times per second.

Very active athletes should be encouraged to have their haemoglobin levels checked fairly frequently, especially if performance or training levels drop or lassitude creeps into their routine. The average haemoglobin for men is 14.7g per 100cm^3 (0.52oz. per 61in^3) of blood and 13.7g per 100cm^3 (0.48oz. per 61in^3) for women. Should the level drop below 12.0g per 100cm^3 (0.42oz. per 61in^3) of blood then a state of anaemia is reached. Both men and women distance runners should expect to have a count of at least 1.0g per 100cm^3 (0.04oz. per 61in^3) of blood higher than this norm. Should the value fall below the norm then a doctor may have to resort to iron injections or to a prescription of a branded iron supplement, together with vitamin C. These preparations, some of which are available without prescriptions, include Ferrograd C, Feospan, ferrous gluconate and ferrous sulphate. The indiscriminate use of iron must be avoided since it increases the viscosity of the blood and so reduces its speed of flow around the body.

The good coach, who is familiar with a particular training group, soon learns to spot the symptoms of approaching anaemia and takes the necessary remedial steps. The tell-tale symptoms are facial skin pallor; unexplained irregularities during training; loss of form; headaches; insomnia; dizziness and so on.

Manganese, zinc and copper are all minerals that aid the function of the enzymes which control many of the metabolic processes within the body. Magnesium has a dual role, not only aiding calcium in the production of bone but also, like chromium, playing a part in energy metabolism (especially in the actions of the hormones glucagon and insulin, which control blood-sugar levels). Iodine has a controlling effect upon the thyroid gland and related hormones. This latter group of trace elements (manganese, zinc, copper, magnesium, chromium and iodine) are only needed in very minute amounts – with a plentiful supply being available in most seafoods.

Sodium and potassium help to control the acid base of the blood. During strenuous and prolonged exercise the body's state becomes more acidic and the homoeostatic response is controlled by these two minerals. However, they are also linked to the electrolyte balance of the body fluid, a proportion of which is lost during exercise in the form of sweat. The body must replace this fluid, but it is unnecessary to replace by supplementing these two minerals (which are also lost during sweating) because the body must be allowed to adapt naturally. A very carefully balanced electrolyte drink may help during prolonged activity in a hot climate but I am of the opinion that water is by far and away the best replacement drink and that to avoid dehydration it should be taken before, during and after very strenuous activity in a hot climate. If water is taken before an event, it must not fill the stomach, nor should it be taken too cold as the system will tend to expel this more quickly. The process of replacing body fluid should start directly after completing the activity, keeping in mind all that has already been said about fluid replacement.

In concluding this chapter I must emphasise that it is not my intention to convey the impression that all vitamins and minerals need to be supplemented artificially. If the diet is sensible and well balanced in every respect, supplementation will not be necessary. However, few of us live in the perfect world.

6

Ergogenic Aids and Supplements

Basically, this term means anything that can aid a working body. Unfortunately, most people now automatically assume that all ergogenic aids have to be drugs. An example of this was highlighted at the 1988 Olympic

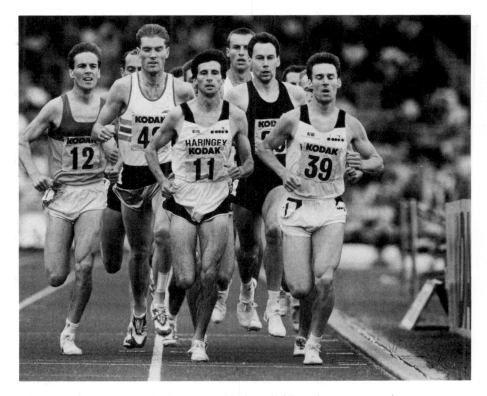

Fig 22   Sebastian Coe leading a world-class field to demonstrate that even this event is no longer the prerogative of the very young.

games in Seoul when Ben Johnson, a Canadian sprinter and 100m world record holder, was stripped of the gold medal for taking anabolic steroids. It is very wrong to assume that drugs are the only way to improve work potential; psychological, climatical and nutritional training programmes can all improve one's capacity.

The rules of most sports are quite specific about drugs and the ergogenic aids which they permit. Certainly, in terms of a very basic philosophy, all of the rules will seem unfair to one group or another. For example, a wealthy sportsperson can afford to train at altitude for an extended period of time while the poorer person might have to resort to blood doping. The end result is the same – an improved oxygen-carrying potential – yet the former is allowed while the latter is illegal.

Modern sport has a problem. Most of its rules (and so its governing philosophy) were established for a society considerably different from the one in which we now live. While some of the rules have been changed to reflect the marching of time the underpinning philosophy is largely that of a bygone era. Sport is now big business, probably one of the largest growth industries of the century. The associated textile, shoe and equipment manufacturers, facility providers and a host of off-shoot industries do not wish to have the clock turned back. The era of commercialism has created a vastly different performer, many of whom look upon sport as a job of work with massive potential earnings. Many amateur philosophers, myself included, believe that sport has taken over from war and that the Olympic arena is now the battlefield. If such a philosophy is correct, then perhaps the rules of war apply – and almost anything goes to support victory. Somewhere between the philosophy of de Coubertin and the above extreme, is one which must set the stage for future generations of sport. It is probably too late to suggest that sport is simply like belonging to an exclusive club, where one has to abide by the rules of the club or leave. Sport must reflect the views of current society but it also has the responsibility to pass on to a future generation a better situation than it inherited. Many people involved with administration at the highest level doubt that our next generation of sportspeople will inherit a better platform for continued improvement. They express concern over the involvement of the entrepreneur, who sees immediate wealth as the objective, rather than showing a concern for the future of the sport.

With such a muddled situation, mainly caused by the rich cash rewards that await those who are successful, it is no wonder that some with a win-at-all-costs philosophy are prepared to cheat: such is the current situation concerning drug abuse among sportspeople. The use of drugs to aid performance in sport is nothing new. In all probability, by means of special diets, the performers at the ancient Greek games were guilty of taking performance-enhancing compounds. In more recent times, the first documentation of drug abuse comes from an Amsterdam canal swim at the turn of the century. Even in those very early days sportspeople were looking for the magic potion – which then included alcohol and nicotine. However, the current situation is vastly more sophisticated and calls for the highest technology in an attempt to detect this level of abuse. The trouble is the 'criminal' (the cheating sportsperson) is always two steps ahead of the 'police' (the dope testers). This situation is unlikely to change very much in the near future.

Types of Drug

It is possible to group the performance-enhancing drugs into ten main categories, all of which have been used in sport to bring about a specific effect, as opposed to simply aiding performance.

Tranquilisers

Tranquilisers are used to calm anxiety, relieve tension and to put the mind at rest without impairing mental functioning. Because of their calming effect they suppress aggression and are therefore of little use to those involved in sports in which they need to be 'fired up'. However, their use in sports such as pistol shooting and archery is well documented.

Local Anaesthetics

Local anaesthetics are widely used in sport, especially in games such as soccer, Rugby, hockey and so on. They are used to 'conceal' an injury by paralysing the sensory nerve endings, so enabling a person to continue in a game without feeling pain. Even the 'freezer spray' roughly fits into this category although longer-lasting anaesthetics need to be injected. Their use can be dangerous since they permit activity on an already injured site, so increasing the likelihood of the injury becoming more serious.

Cardiac Stimulants

Cardiac stimulants are used to bring about an increased cardiac output by affecting the force of contraction of the heart. They improve the circulation to all of the vital organs, in particular the liver, which in turn improves the provision of energy at most levels of exercise. Their immediate use would appear to be in the short-duration events. I have never come across their use in sport, although such drugs have been detected in sportspeople.

Cardiac Depressants

The opposite of cardiac stimulants, depressants are used to decrease the functioning of the heart during training so that it is much harder to work. When the body is relieved of the depressant, just prior to competition, a so-called 'supercharged' effect is experienced.

Anti-Parkinsonian Drugs

Such drugs are used in the treatment of Parkinson's disease, in which sufferers find it hard to initiate and control movements because of loss of muscle tone. The vibrating teacup is a recognisable symptom of the disease. With this drug a fair degree of control is achievable, reducing muscular rigidity and giving improved balance and motor co-ordination; this could certainly be of value to a person who is already controlled but would like 'that little bit extra'.

CNS Stimulants

CNS stimulants are responsible for the death of at least one sportsman. They form the amphetamine-cocaine group and work in a manner similar to adrenaline – that is by preparing the body to fight. They produce an indifference to fatigue, giving the performer a sense of 'Dutch courage'. Linked closely to the group are drugs such as adrenaline, ephedrine and pseudo-ephedrine, all of which now find themselves on the banned list of substances. An unfortunate side-effect of this is that it is now difficult to prescribe many of the simple cough and decongestant remedies during competition.

CNS Depressants

This group has already been mentioned under the heading of cardiac depressants but they are also depressants of the central nervous system, otherwise known as beta blockers. It has been suggested that athletes use these drugs to control the flow of adrenaline so that they can consciously channel all their resources into a single explosive effort. In all probability, taking these drugs avoids the lethargic state which nature uses to combat the uncontrolled flow of adrenaline.

Vasodilators

Vasodilators improve the blood supply to both cardiac and skeletal muscle. Their use might seem obvious to the layman for the short term, but over the long term they can bring about the opposite response – mainly due to nature's homoeostatic effects. While these drugs are very uncommon in sport, samples have been discovered, suggesting that sportspeople have used them.

Synthetic Steroids

This group fits into two very distinct categories so far as sport is concerned: legal and illegal. The legal group includes the birth-control pill, which is used to control the menstruation of women competitors. They are used very effectively in sport to ensure that pre-menstrual tension (PMT) does not occur just before a major competition. However, even this well-tried pill is not without side-effects, one of which is to reduce vitamin C levels (others include fluid retention, weight gain and psychological disturbances with tremendous mood variations). The side-effects vary considerably from person to person and from prescribed pill to pill.

The illegal group, which form the anabolics and the androgens, have probably had more effect upon sport – in terms of enhancing perform-ances – than any of the other so-called ergogenic aids. Sportspeople, and in particular those from the power-based sports, 'stack' (take combina-tions of drugs) in order to take advantage of both the anabolic (building up) and androgenic (masculine) effects, depending upon their particular phase of training. In spite of all of the elaborate testing techniques used to detect the presence of these drugs, many sportspeople adopt a very sophisticated and informed approach to this unfortunate aspect of modern sport. The various substances are phased carefully throughout the year so that the most anabolic (easily detected) drugs are used during the strength-promoting phases and the less detectable drugs are used closer to the competition period, when testing is more likely.

It must be accepted that the anabolic steroid is *not* a magic pill which is simply popped in before competition. It is a preparation that has to be wilfully taken during training. The steroid does not automatically do anything but, through a gluco-corticoid effect, it increases one's work capacity by permitting a faster and more efficient recovery from the stress of training. The euphoric effect also produced by steroids and associated with an androgen response is used to good advantage in sport.

The presence of the human growth hormone (HCG) has also been detected in a fairly wide spectrum of sportspeople, suggesting that even this avenue is being used to improve performance. The ideas and applications in this area are almost endless – but not without serious side-effects. At the time of writing, sport has a major problem in the thriving black-market industry for steroids. As the law now stands it is not illegal to possess anabolic steroids, indeed they can be purchased over the counter in most European countries. However, it looks as if different legislation might soon be introduced.

Some researchers have claimed that anabolic steroids do not work. If these people had to work at the 'sharp end' of sport they would realise that their effect upon power-based performances is dramatic and that they have improved certain records by up to fifteen per cent, mainly through significant increases in strength levels.

Blocking Agents

Blocking agents, some of which are diuretics, can mask the presence of another drug, such as the steroid group, in a urine sample which might otherwise have proven positive. Drugs such as probenicid, which has this property, are now included on the banned list by most organising bodies.

Blood Doping

Technically, blood doping cannot be termed drug taking. It involves taking blood from a performer, separating out the red blood-cells and then returning the packed red cells to the original donor at a later date. The doping must be done under totally sterile conditions, especially during refrigeration (the period before the cells are transfused). There is some evidence to support the belief that there has been at least one death due to blood doping and that there are a number of incidents of quite serious bacterial infections, including hepatitis, resulting from this method of cheating.

Once the transfusion has taken place the receiver will have a consider-ably enhanced oxygen-carrying potential due to the extra red blood-cells circulating in the body. The situation is fairly short-lived as the homo-eostatic action of the body soon establishes the status quo.

The inclusion of a chapter, mainly on drugs, within a text on nutrition might at first sight seem questionable. It is my opinion that the situation is a very serious problem and it is essential that action is taken to remedy the present state of affairs. However, there is also the difficulty of knowing exactly where to draw the line between what constitutes a drug as an ergogenic aid and what does not. For example, in certain nations in the world vitamin B_{15} is simply that – a vitamin – while in others it is considered a drug.

Supplementation

This is probably one of the most controversial aspects of nutrition. It has its devotees who verge on the fanatical and it also has its staunchest opponents, many of them from the medical profession. Food supplementation is precisely what it says: an aid – and not a replacement – to a good diet. Eating from a wide variety of food, containing a good balance of all of the nutrients, vitamins and minerals will mean supplementation of food is not really necessary. However, many people in society do not eat correctly, and so supplementation may be the only alternative.

Many sports remain the prerogative of the young. This group of people, a good proportion of them being students, have probably taken themselves away from mother's home cooking. Too frequently they have to rely upon mass catering, convenience or 'junk' food as their only source of nutrients. A survey of student sportspeople carried out in 1985 indicated some very alarming facts, particularly among the young female sample. The largest proportion of this group did not eat any fresh vegetables from one week to the next; indeed a number existed on chocolate bars and tuna fish sandwiches. It is obvious that these people are in very real danger of having a diet inadequate for their needs.

It is mind-boggling to read through a list of substances produced by most health-food companies. Indeed, if people took all of the products in the recommended dose, they would be forced to spend the largest proportion of the day popping pills (or the equivalent) into their mouths. The extensive range starts at alpha-alpha and runs through to zinc with almost every letter of the alphabet covered. Of course it would be doing the health-food companies a terrible disservice to suggest that it is their intention to encourage people to take all their products all the time. Most of the people in the trade are totally ethical, but at the same time catering for any specific nutritional whim the customer may care to have.

The origins of food supplements (and so the health-food trade) dates back centuries, the forerunner probably being the herbalist. Indeed, quite a number of the current preparations are still steeped in the mystique of the ancient apothecary. Many of them are well-proven formulae which have stood the test of time, with a particular favourite being passed down from generation to generation.

I am a firm believer in supplementing the diet, but there must be certain reservations. The first is that supplements must never replace a good, healthy, mixed diet. I tend to regard them more as an insurance policy against any possibility of the diet being unable to provide the necessary nutrients. The food supplements taken must vary from person to person and from sport to sport. Sportspeople need to look at their needs, carefully examine whether or not their diet caters for these needs and then supplement with the appropriate substances. When making a critical examination it should be remembered that refined, processed, frozen and heat-treated foods do not necessarily contain the level of nutrients found in the raw materials.

It is almost certain that supplementation of the three basic nutrients will be unnecessary, as almost any diet will contain enough of these. However, in most of the power-based sports I do advocate the use of amino acids in the free form. Other than this we are left with vitamins, minerals and the odd trace element, together with a few other substances that might be necessary for a particular individual.

Vitamin A

As this is a fat-soluble vitamin there should be no need to supplement unless the diet is lacking in dairy products, fish and eggs.

Vitamin B

This group is worth supplementing since it is a very large group and has many complex actions of vital importance to the sportsperson. As it is a water-soluble vitamin there are no fears of it becoming toxic since any surplus is simply secreted in the urine. This is quite an important complex to supplement, especially where refined flour is used for breadmaking. It is also quite plentiful in most red meats especially those classed as offal.

Vitamin C

This is probably the most fragile of the vitamins, being partially or wholly destroyed by any form of storage, preserving or cooking. It is required in fairly large amounts and as a water-soluble vitamin its life span in the body is restricted. Those people who do not eat fruit and vegetables are certainly quite likely to be deficient. I always recommend that most of my athletes supplement this vitamin when I sense that they are low or run down. A supplement of 1g per day should ensure that the person is not short of this most important vitamin.

Vitamin D

This vitamin is formed by the skin through the action of sunlight, although a form of the vitamin is found in fish-liver oils and in eggs. While this vitamin cannot really be supplemented I am a firm believer in the effects of full-spectrum lighting (i.e. lighting which mimics the rays of the sun). Dr Damien Downing of the York nutritional clinic, in his book *Let there be Light*, emphasises the many advantages of therapy with full-spectrum lighting. It is mainly used as a treatment for stress-related illnesses, but there are claims that it can also increase oxygen uptake, make more glycogen available and increase testosterone levels by over twenty per cent. This research is very exciting and it could be the power-based sportsperson's answer to anabolic steroids. Full-spectrum lighting must not be confused with a sunbed, since this only radiates a very narrow spectrum which could prove harmful.

Vitamin E

This is a very important vitamin for the sportsperson and those who do not include wheat-germ, vegetable oil, whole-meal bread and eggs in their diet must consider supplementation. It is a fat-soluble vitamin and can prove toxic in large amounts.

Essential Polyunsaturated Fatty Acids (PUFAs)

These are essential in the diet as they keep cells in a state of efficiency and help to produce prostaglandins, which have a considerable effect upon many of the body functions; they are present in most seed oils. Those athletes, particularly the very thin distance-runners who try to exclude most forms of fat from their diet, would do well to supplement these. Frequently linked in with this group is a substance known as lecithin. In Chapter 1 I made specific reference to its action within the body. For certain sports and at certain times lecithin supplementation may also enhance performance.

Minerals

Calcium
Calcium is essential for sportspeople, particularly women who can lose vast quantities during certain times of their life. The recommended daily intake is about 1g. Those who exclude dairy products from their diet must supplement.

Chromium
Chromium is another mineral essential for those involved in sport as it has a very significant effect upon growth and energy levels through its association with the liver and the conversion of fats to energy. It also has an effect upon the immune system. The recommended daily intake should be in the region of 200µg. I recommend the supplementation of this through brewers' yeast (which also provides much of the B complex of vitamins).

Iodine
This is essential for a healthy heart and for the correct absorption of proteins, so the sportsperson must not be low in iodine. The recommended daily intake is about 500µg and I recommend supplementing it through kelp.

Iron
This mineral is essential to the body, is quite likely to need supplementation and causes concern to many people in sport, particularly women and those involved in endurance events. Iron is present in offal and certain green vegetables, although it must be stressed that iron from a vegetable source is not absorbed well by the body. As already stated earlier in the text, too much iron can affect the viscocity (speed of circulation) of the blood. Periodic supplementation of iron can only be beneficial . If this is supported by regular blood tests this is an extra bonus.

Magnesium
Since magnesium serves as a co-enzyme in the production of ATP sportspeople need a good supply of this mineral. The recommended

daily intake for sportspeople is about 1,000mg. It is present in all green leafy vegetables so those who avoid these must supplement.

Manganese

Manganese helps with energy, growth and muscle efficiency, together with an effect on vitamin C levels. It is present in a wide variety of foods, especially nuts, but it is worth supplementing through a good multi-mineral product.

Selenium

Selenium is essential for working at peak efficiency. It is very hard to obtain from most natural sources so a supplement through a multi-mineral will cater for all needs.

Zinc

Zinc is available in many foods so there should be no problem obtaining sufficient quantities. However, many of our nutritional habits, such as drinking tea and coffee, reduce its availability. Because it plays a vital role in hormone production, in particular the sex hormones, it is very important that the sportsperson who avoids offal and who drinks tea or coffee should consider supplementation. Moreover, women on the birth-control pill would be well advised to heed this advice.

Most of the vitamins and minerals are available in multi-mineral or multi-vitamin form. This is probably the best way of taking them as it avoids taking too many pill supplements. However, the levels available in most of the multi-forms may not necessarily be adequate for special therapy. In such cases the person should look towards an individual supplement which will normally be available. One point is certain: a very small investment in a multi-mineral or multi-vitamin supplement will, in the end, prove a very cheap insurance policy.

As far as supplementation is concerned, this only leaves the highly controversial topic of amino acids. The whole field of what specific amino acids do for the body is complex and understanding is continually changing. At present, amino-acid therapy is the vogue for many of the leading sportspeople in the world. There is also a wealth of research material now becoming available supporting the use of **argenine** and **ornithine** in particular. I would certainly recommend the supplementation of these two, although a general, free-form amino-acid supplement would be an added precautionary measure.

7

Alcohol, Tobacco
and Sleep

Many people might be surprised to see these three topics included in a text on nutrition since only alcohol can be termed a beverage, so having a direct link with nutrition. However, smoking does affect the availability of certain nutrients and timing one's eating with regard to sleeping is something the sportsperson has to consider.

Alcohol

Many of the major sports played throughout the United Kingdom (such as both codes of Rugby, soccer, hockey and cricket) are frequently called the social sports and certainly social drinking forms a major part of the club's existence. Indeed, many clubs can only survive because of the bar revenue and consequently many of the sponsors of these sports are breweries. While the consumption of alcohol cannot usually be classed as excessive among sportspeople, there is no doubt that society in general has a problem which it must soon face if the general health of our youth is not to deteriorate. Indeed many very influential people, particularly from sport, are already putting to our youth an alternative health style.

In terms of nutrition, alcohol is very high in energy. However, in order for this to be utilised it must undergo a very slow process in the liver which initially converts the alcohol to fat – so entering the energy cycle at a later stage. It is for these reasons that alcohol affects the health of the liver and is termed 'dead calories'. There is some evidence to suggest that there is a link between depleting levels of both vitamin C and vitamin B with alcohol. Even if for no other reason, the view of the teetotal athlete can be supported.

Alcohol is a proven diuretic and as such can cause dehydration. It certainly impairs motor function, although I must admit that I have never

81

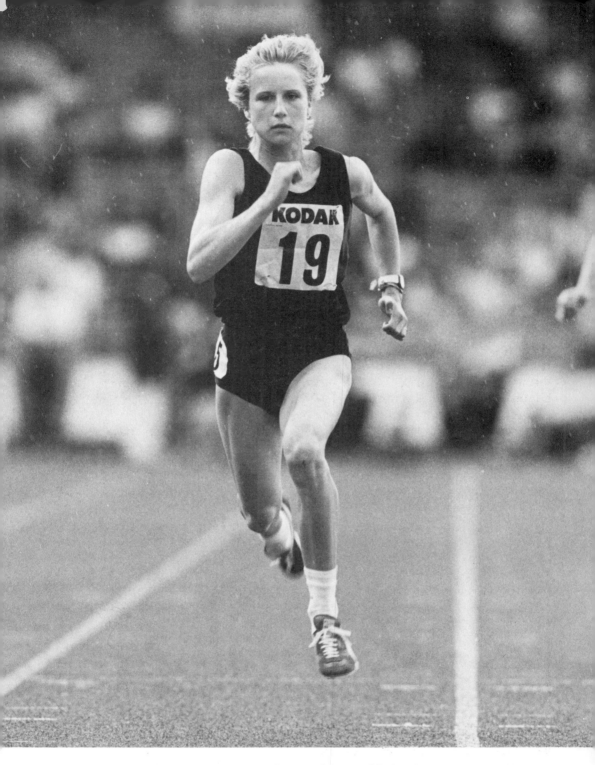

Fig 23   Katherine Merry, currently one of the world's brightest sprinting prospects. Can nurture take over when nature contributes less?

seen an elite sportsman take to the field in an intoxicated state! However, there are rumours that good cricketers have survived the immediate post-lunch overs not in total control of all of their faculties and the local Saturday afternoon game is not without similar incidences. Alcohol also reduces one's aerobic capacity and decreases the contractile state of skeletal muscle. Hence my advice to anyone who wishes to aspire to a good performance level is to keep on the side of moderation as far as alcohol is concerned.

Tobacco

Tobacco contains drugs that undoubtedly have a very profound effect upon the health of our nation and pro rata certainly accounts for more deaths than any of the ergogenic aids used in sport. There is, accordingly, legislation banning drugs in sport – yet this lethal substance is allowed to continue in society unlimited. Would this be the case if it were not a prime source of income for the government?

In terms of nutrition there is only a very tenuous link between nicotine and levels of vitamin B and C. It would also be very unwise, in a text of this nature, not to highlight the effects which it has upon oxygen uptake and breathing. I can only insist that it is a disgusting habit which has nothing at all to redeem its antisocial nature.

Sleep

No one can participate in sport at a high level and not have adequate rest. It is a good adage for the sportsperson to consider that 'one hour before midnight is worth at least two after'. The time of sleeping can and does considerably influence diet. There should be a period of at least two hours between eating and retiring to bed. Failure to observe this simple fact could, over a long term, produce a serious illness.

Research workers in Finland suggest that the best to time to use amino-acid therapy is at night. The theory is that any rebuilding process takes place at this time and there is protein available for this function. However, my own personal observations indicate that both amino-acid and vitamin B supplementation produces a degree of insomnia and should be used well in advance of retiring to bed.

There is evidence to suggest that those who wish to lose weight should exercise first thing in the morning before eating. Here the theory relates to the availability of glycogen – the simple energy provider. In the morning glycogen reserves are very low so energy is provided by utilising fats.

The main object of this brief chapter has been to help create an awareness of the three factors rather than supply a list of pseudo-scientific facts. Sport demands a healthy life-style and these three aspects certainly have an effect upon that.

8

Dietary Considerations for Individual-Based Sports

Introduction

In this section it is my intention to illustrate how energy levels can be calculated (I have actually taken my examples, where applicable, from the handbook accompanying the 1988 Olympic games). In this handbook all of the competitors are listed in event categories, giving their heights, weights and ages. The individual nations' handbooks give employment categories for their competitors. Where the chosen sport is not from the Olympic list, I have taken examples from top-class performers who are known to me. I have obtained the various training loads from international-status coaches of the individual sports. The examples selected therefore represent a true picture of those involved in their various sports.

The suggested daily menus, designed to cater for the various energy-expenditure levels will be found in Chapter 13, together with special diets such as carbohydrate loading. This system has been selected to avoid too much repetition. I have also avoided using diets which I think might be impractical for the sportsperson. The foods included are all typical of what sportspeople eat at major competitions. I have avoided the idea of a need to convert everyone on to a 'health nut' menu.

It is sensible to mention once again those factors which influence the calculation of energy requirements, which are:

the basal rate (A) which is mainly influenced by weight and to a lesser degree by gender, height and age
the basic chores of life and work (B)
the energy involved in the practising of one's sport (C)

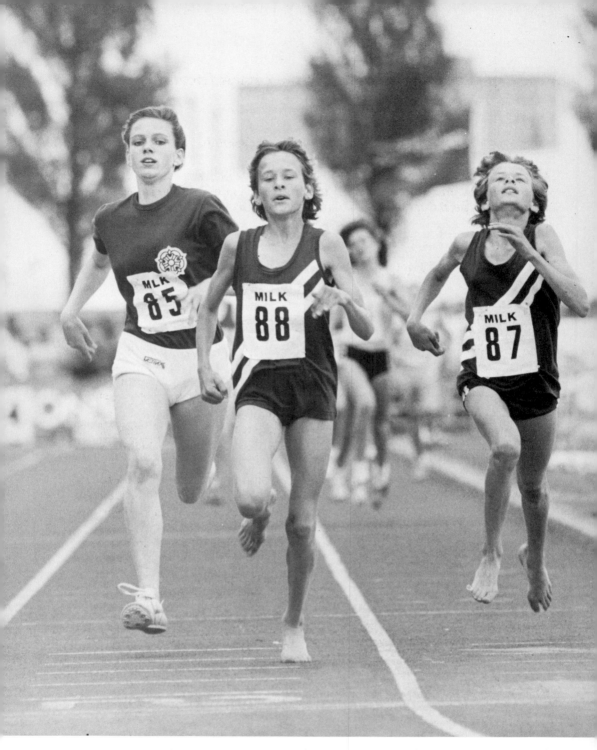

Fig 24   The young Tulloch twins, whose parents were also good runners, illustrate how food products (in this case milk) like to be associated with fitness.

$$A + B + C = total\ energy\ requirements$$

This total should equal that of the ingested food – where there is a large discrepancy then the efficiency of the body will be greatly impeded. It must be accepted that there may be an error in calculation of the order of ten per cent.

Dietary Considerations

1. Female, 20 years old
Height: 168cm (5ft 6in)
Weight: 59kg (130lb)
Occupation: typist
Event: sprinting

Basal rate	1,380kcal
Occupation + chores allowance (=50%)	690kcal
Training (jogging 10min, stretching 15min, 6 × 120m flat out, standing, walking between exercises)	806kcal
Total (per day)	2,876kcal

In order to achieve an energy balance the woman listed would need to eat food to the energy equivalent of 2,800–3,000kcal per day. Such an allowance would also suffice if she were a sprint hurdler, whereas a 400m hurdler would need an increase of about ten per cent. A male sprinter of similar height and weight as this requires 3,500–3,700kcal per day.

2. Male, 25 years old
Height: 183cm (6ft)
Weight: 70kg (150lb)
Occupation: motor mechanic
Event: long jump

Basal rate	1,450kcal
Occupation + chores allowance (=70%)	1,015kcal
Training (jogging 10min, stretching 15min, 10 × full effort jumps, 6 × 50m sprints, recovery activity)	1,270kcal
Total (per day)	3,735kcal

For an energy balance the above long jumper would require 3,500–4,0000kcal per day. A typical woman in the same event would require approximately 3,000kcal per day.

3.   Male, 25 years old
Height: 188cm (6ft 2in)
Weight: 100kg (220lb)
Occupation: labourer
Event: heavy throwing

Basal rate	1,900kcal
Occupation + chores allowance (=100%)	1,900kcal
Training (jogging 10min, stretching and throwing 30min, weight-lifting 1hr)	2,180kcal
Total (per day)	5,980kcal

The above thrower would require food equivalent of approximately 6,000kcal per day. A typical woman in the same event, with the same level of training, would require about 5,000kcal per day.

4.   Female, 20 years old
Height: 168cm (5ft 6in)
Occupation: housewife
Event: marathon

Basal rate	1,225kcal
Occupation + chores allowance (=70%)	856kcal
Training (running 40min a.m., running 40min p.m.)	1,600kcal
Total (per day)	3,681kcal

5.   Female, 16 years old
Height: 168cm (5ft 6in)
Weight: 54kg (120lb)
Occupation: schoolgirl
Event: swimming

Basal rate	1,320kcal
Occupation + chores allowance (=50%)	660kcal
Training (70 × 50m at 70m/min)	1,600kcal
Total (per day)	3,580kcal

6.   Male, 23 years old
Height: 183cm (6ft)
Weight: 78kg (172lb)
Occupation: PE teacher
Event: swimming

Basal rate	1,700kcal
Occupation + chores allowance (=70%)	1,190kcal

Training (mixed distances and speeds, averaging 70m/min)   1,840kcal
Total (per day)   4,730kcal

Examples 5 and 6 are based on routines used by top-class swimmers. The volume of their work is impressive and accounts for the high energy expenditure. It must also be accepted that many swimmers do two or more training sessions each day. This would have to be added to the above figures.

7.   Female, 16 years old
Height: 168cm (5ft 6in)
Weight: 54kg (120lb)
Occupation: schoolgirl
Event: gymnastics
   Basal rate   1,320kcal
   Occupation + chores allowance (=50%)   660kcal
   Training (mixed floor work and vaulting 2hr)   1,150kcal
   Total (per day)   3,130kcal

It can be very difficult to calculate the energy expenditure of a gymnast because sessions may include much time devoted to skill practice, as well as lengthy periods of analysis and discussion with the coach. The nature of the work, except for the asymmetric bars, is of short duration and intermittent. On a day which includes asymmetric-bar work an extra ten per cent should be added, producing a figure in the region of 3,550kcal per day.

8.   Male, 25 years old
Height: 178cm (5ft 10in)
Weight: 73kg (160lb)
Occupation: salesman
Event: gymnastics
   Basal rate   1,640kcal
   Occupation + chores allowance (=60%)   984kcal
   Training (high bar, pommel horse 2hr)   1,368kcal
   Total (per day)   3,992kcal

9.   Male, 25 years old
Height: 183cm (6ft)
Weight: 78kg (170lb)
Occupation: motor mechanic

Event: distance cycling

Basal rate	1,700kcal
Occupation + chores allowance (=70%)	1,190kcal
Training (4hr at 12mph)	2,880kcal
Total (per day)	5,770kcal

Some research done on cyclists established that a distance cyclist needed between 80 and 87kcal/kg of body-weight per day. Taking the lower figure of 80kcal/kg per day the above man would require 6,240kcal per day, there being a difference of 500kcal between the two methods of calculation. This is still within the ten per cent margin of error associated with calculations of this nature.

Readers should now reter to Chapter 13 where the typical menus for differing energy requirements are detailed.

9
Dietary Considerations for Major Team Games

In this chapter the major team games played in the United Kingdom are examined. Since this text is intended as much for the élite player as for the average club player, examples are taken from professional players belonging to the clubs such as Liverpool and Leeds United football clubs. The full-time professional player is in a situation unlike amateurs since playing and training is his or her job of work and many clubs train for four

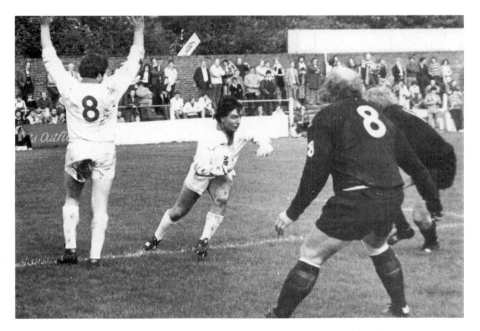

Fig 25   The New Zealand number eight forward waits to tackle the opposing back; note the differences in physique and age between backs and forwards.

hours or more each day. However, my observations have indicated that, in the end, there is not a great deal of difference between the training methods of the very good amateur and the professional sides. What difference there is can be whittled down, essentially, to the number of hours per day spent training.

Because of the different nature of the team games I have used a different form for the dietary calculations (based once more on the work of Professor N.N. Yakovlev). He worked with top international players and produced a table which gave the total number of kilocalories such sportsmen required and also analysed the part played in this total amount by the three main nutrients. These calculations include all the daily chores, training routines and so on. As with the other method, body-weight is the significant factor.

1.   Male, 25 years old
Height: 178cm (5ft 10in)
Weight: 70kg (154lb)
Occupation: professional footballer
    Daily energy requirements: 63–67kcal/kg/day
    Using the mean value (65kcal/kg/day) this becomes:
        $65 \times 70 = 4,550$ kcal per day
    A heavier player of 82kg (180lb) needs:
        $65 \times 82 = 5,330$ kcal per day

Speaking in very general terms the average full-time professional soccer player should be able to keep a lean body consuming in the region of 4,500–5,500kcal per day. This would probably need to be reduced on a match day when the volume of work would, of course, be restricted to ninety minutes only (although the intensity of activity should be higher).

Most of the research which has been carried out on sport and nutrition has been performed either in Russia or the United States, where Rugby is not played. It would be very convenient to say that it is a cross between American football and soccer and that by this method approximate values could be obtained. However, as part of my work with a top-class Rugby league team I have done many game analyses to calculate how far an individual player sprints, how many tackles he makes and so on, during a typical game. Hence I intend to base my work for this sport on these analyses. As there is a considerable difference in weight between a typical forward and a typical back, I have made allowances for this in my calculations. I have also selected specific training patterns from my own training plans with international-class players.

2. **Activity**

	Forward kcal/day	Back kcal/day
Training day 1		
basal rate	1,800	1,500
occupation + chores	1,800	1,500
jogging for 10min	180	130
sprint/walk for 10min	900	750
ball work for 30 min	450	380
Total	5,130	4,260
Training day 2		
basal rate + chores	3,600	3,000
jogging for 10min	180	130
callisthenics for 10min	100	80
weight-training for 20min	800	600
recovery activity during weights	70	60
Total	4,750	3,870
Game day		
basal rate + activities	3,600	3,000
game	1,100	900
Total	4,700	3,900

3. Female, 20 years old
Height: 178cm (5ft 10in)
Weight: 64kg (140lb)
Occupation: PE teacher
Event: field hockey

Basal rate	1,460kcal
Occupation + chores allowance (=70%)	1,022kcal
Training: callisthenics 15min	75kcal
sprint/walk/jog 10min	510kcal
ball work 30min	320kcal
Total (per day)	3,387kcal

On a match day the requirement would be 3,969kcal per day. Hence, the above player should be able to keep a good energy balance with between 3,000 and 4,000kcal each day. My recommendation would be to keep alternate days, one devoted to the lower intake and the next to the higher intake.

4.   Male, 25 years old
Height: 183cm (6ft)
Weight: 78kg (172lb)
Occupation: accountant
Event: field hockey

Basal rate	1,700kcal
Occupation + chores allowance (=50%)	850kcal
Training: callisthenics 15min	95kcal
sprints 10min	580kcal
ball work 30min	380kcal
Total (per day)	3,605kcal

On a match day, the modified norms of Yakovlev should now be increased by about 1,000kcal, so the value would increase to 4,600kcal or so per day. Hence, as was the case with the female player a good balance can be achieved with a diet supplying a daily equivalent of between 3,600 and 4,600kcal.

It is interesting to note that Yakovlev gives an identical allowance, in terms of basic nutrients and daily calorie intake, to both basketball and volleyball. Hence any variation in the daily requirements for these two sports will come solely through the influence of the basal rate and the occupation allowance.

5.   Male, 25 years old
Height: 193cm (6ft 4in)
Weight: 86kg (190lb)
Occupation: PE teacher
Event: basketball

Basal rate	1,900kcal
Occupation + chores allowance (=70%)	1,330kcal
Training: skill work 80min evenings	840kcal
Total (per day)	4,070kcal

For the full-time professional player (using the norms presented by Yakovlev) the value would increase to 5,332kcal per day. Hence, with the accepted degree of accuracy, the tall basketball or volleyball player could achieve an energy balance with a diet supplying between 4,000 and 5,000kcal per day.

Netball is largely restricted to countries of the British Commonwealth; it is very popular in Great Britain, almost a national sport for women in New Zealand and is popular in both Australia and the West Indies. Some Western and Eastern European countries play the game up to international level, while in most other countries it remains a game for schoolgirls. Because of this, the research work available does not include netball as one of the analysed games. Although similar to basketball, the tempo of the game is considerably slower, particularly when the player is in contact with the ball. The game is a combination of: short sprints by which the player runs into a position to receive the ball; a slower, almost continuous, activity as part of the defensive play; and jumping to receive or intercept the ball. Hence, by analysing the movement of a player during a game, it is possible to arrive at a fairly accurate figure for a specific position as part of a game. When netball players are observed in training, their routines are very similar to those for the other major games in that they train for endurance (both strength and speed), pure speed and power, and skill.

6.   Female, 25 year old
Height: 175cm (5ft 9in)
Weight: 66kg (147lb)
Occupation: PE teacher
Event: netball (centre court player)

Basal rate	1,440kcal
Occupation + chores allowance (=70%)	1,008kcal
Training: jogging 10min	252kcal
stretching for mobility 10min	65kcal
10 × 30m sprint and recovery	200kcal
circuit training 20min	310kcal
skill game 20min	180kcal
Total (per day)	3,455kcal

The above example represents a very typical training session for an international-class player. A game analysis reveals that in the course of a county-level game the player requires only about 3,000kcal to keep the energy balance. Therefore, a diet supplying between 3,000 and 3,500kcal should assure that not too much adipose tissue is deposited about the body.

95

10

Dietary Considerations for the Martial Arts

In this chapter the sports of boxing, wrestling, judo and fencing are considered. I appreciate that there are a whole host of Oriental martial arts such as karate and aikido but these are beyond the scope of this text. Boxing and wrestling, in particular, present a complicated situation as both have professional versions which usually last considerably longer than their amateur equivalents. Also, both of these sports have weight categories which vary from under 51kg (112lb) to the super heavyweight category which is open.

1. Male, 25 years old
Height: 157cm (5ft 2in)
Weight: 48kg (106lb)
Occupation: labourer
Event: light flyweight boxing

Basal rate	1,300kcal
Occupation + chores allowance (=100%)	1,300kcal
Training: jogging/running 30min	600kcal
5 × 3min continuous skipping	450kcal
6 × 3min sparring/shadow boxing	180kcal
medicine-ball work	280kcal
Total (per day)	4,110kcal

Using the above example, the very light boxer performing the typical training load requires 4,170kcal per day, which should avoid any weight increase – a prime concern for all boxers.

An alternative way of making the calculations would be based on the norms produced by Yakovlev. Using these norms given by Yakovlev the boxer has an energy requirement of 65–70kcal/kg per day. In this situation, the flyweight has an energy requirement of 3,360kcal per day

Weight category	Weight		Daily energy expenditure	Percentage increase in energy expenditure
	(kg)	[lb]	(kcal)	
flyweight	51.0	[112]	4,370	5
bantamweight	54.0	[119]	4,570	10
featherweight	57.0	[126]	4,770	15
lightweight	60.0	[132]	4,980	20
light welterweight	63.5	[140]	5,190	25
welterweight	67.0	[148]	5,300	30
light middleweight	71.0	[157]	5,500	35
middleweight	75.0	[165]	5,700	40
light heavyweight	81.0	[165]	5,900	45
heavyweight	91.0	[201]	6,100	55
super heavyweight	>91.0	[>201]	>6,100	>55

Fig 26   The percentage increase in energy expenditure – above those values given for a light flyweight, above – for other weight categories. These values assume a proportional increase in height from one weight category to the next.

while the heavyweight requires 5,750kcal per day. Both methods should ensure that the boxer keeps within his weight limits.

There are several similarities between boxing and wrestling, the major one for our purposes being that both have weight categories. However, even the most casual observer would instantly recognise a difference in size (especially at the heavyweight end of the scale). At Olympic level there are two recognised versions of the sport, Greco–Roman and freestyle. Despite this complication I intend to treat the sport simply as 'wrestling' and use the Yakovlev system for calculating the daily energy requirements.

Weight		kcal/day
(kg)	(lb)	
52	114	3,536
57	125	3,876
63	139	4,284
70	154	4,760
78	172	5,304
87	191	5,916
97	213	6,596

Fig 27   The daily energy requirements for boxers of differing weights.

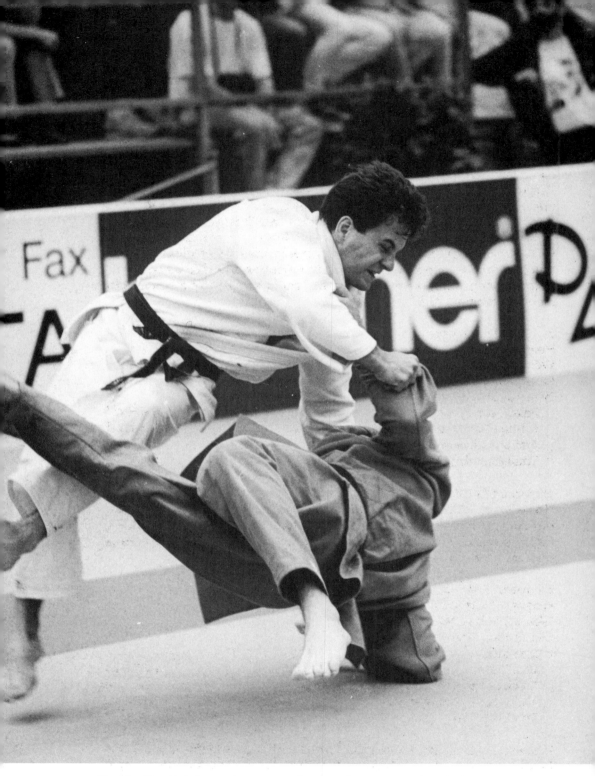

Fig 28   *Physical demands are great in a combat sport such as judo.*

It must be accepted that Fig 27 is based upon a typical training (or competition) day for a top-class performer and so it includes all of the chore and training variables which are part of this method of calculation. The chart also emphasises the extreme effect which weight can have upon the energy requirements of an individual.

It has been difficult to decide which of the Oriental combat arts to include in this section. I have been influenced in my choice mainly through the co-operation of a judo coach who has allowed me to observe training sessions and so work out the competition and training patterns. Judo is a popular sport throughout the world and is practised by both men and women.

2. Female, 23 years old
Height: 177cm (5ft 10in)
Weight: 73kg (160lb)
Occupation: secretary
Event: judo

Basal rate	1,525kcal
Occupation + chores allowance (=50%)	763kcal
Training: intermittent skills 2hr	771kcal
Total (per day)	3,059kcal

This value (3,059kcal) would be roughly the same for a competition day. However, it will be affected both by the number of competitions and the duration of each contest. Assuming that a contest lasts about fifteen minutes the above person is likely to expend about 214kcal of energy during its course.

3. Male, 35 years old
Height: 183cm (6ft)
Weight: 90kg (198lb)
Occupation: banker
Event: judo

Basal rate	1,815kcal
Occupation + chores allowance (=50%)	907kcal
Training: intermittent skills 2hr	970kcal
Total (per day)	3,692kcal

In competition (and assuming a bout duration of fifteen minutes) this judoka would require 253kcal to fuel the energy expended in a single contest.

4. Male, 32 years old
Height: 183cm (6ft)
Weight: 75kg (178lb)
Occupation: stockbroker
Event: fencing (sabre)

Basal rate	1,640kcal
Occupation + chores allowance (=50%)	820kcal
Training; intermittent skills 2hr	825kcal
Total (per cent)	3,285kcal

5. Female, 29 years old
Height; 169cm (5ft 7in)
Weight: 60kg (132lb)
Occupation: librarian
Event: fencing (foil)

Basal rate	1,360kcal
Occupation + chores allowance (=50%)	680kcal
Training: intermittent skills 2hr	558kcal
Total (per day)	2,598kcal

Those fencers who train at other activities for speed, strength and endurance should make reference to the equivalent sections for athletes in Chapter 8 in order to calculate the energy requirements necessary for a particular training session. However, it is unlikely that their basic requirements will rise much above the 3,500kcal per day given for the fencer.

11

Dietary Considerations for Racquet Sports

It is in the field of racquet sports, and tennis in particular, that the gulf between the professional circuit player and the amateur enthusiast is especially wide. Also, at the very top level much can depend upon the draw, for a game may be over in three straight sets or on the other hand last more than four hours. It is also common knowledge, mainly through the Press, that many of the top-flight tennis players actually warm up for several hours before competing in a tournament match. This may mean playing for a period in the region of five hours with only very short breaks for recovery.

It can be calculated that any player who follows such a routine would need in the region of 3,300kcal to fuel the tennis alone. This figure should be increased by at least ten per cent for the bigger, heavier player. Hence, it seems most likely that the average professional circuit player, on a match day, is likely to require in excess of 5,000kcal to keep the energy balance. The person who wishes to play the game for fun seems a long way removed from this situation. Hence the following examples will be taken from those who wish to play the game socially at their local club.

1. Female, 23 years old
Height: 177cm (5ft 10in)
Weight: 68kg (150lb)
Occupation: housewife
Event: tennis

Basal rate	1,480kcal
Occupation + chores allowance (=70%)	1,036kcal
Competition tennis 2hr	1,452kcal
Total (per day)	3,968kcal

2.   Male, 50 years old
Height: 183cm (6ft)
Weight: 95kg (210lb)
Occupation: company director
Event: tennis

Basal rate	1,855kcal
Occupation + chores allowance (=50%)	927kcal
Social tennis 2hr	600kcal
Total (per day)	3,382kcal

3.   Male, 35 years old
Height: 188cm (6ft 2in)
Weight: 91kg (200lb)
Occupation: architect/valuer
Event: squash

Basal rate	1,800kcal
Occupation + chores allowance (=70%)	1,260kcal
Squash 45min	540kcal
Total (per day)	3,600kcal

Like tennis there is a vast difference between the social keep-fit squash player who fits in a thirty-minute game between business appointments and the professional tournament player who will be on the court several hours each day.

   In the case of the professional, playing a high-quality, fast game, the energy expenditure is in the region of 250–350kcal per game, depending upon the physique of the player. Hence, a quick calculation can be made for the tournament player who seeks this level of perfection. However, the majority of people who play the game fit into the category of social players, some of whom wish to progress up the club ladder while others simply wish to have a quick thrash around the court as part of keeping fit.

4.   Female, 26 years old
Height: 157cm (5ft 2in)
Weight: 57kg (126lb)
Occupation: PE teacher
Event: squash

Basal rate	1,320kcal
Occupation + chores allowance (=70%)	924kcal
Squash 45min	450kcal
Total (per day)	2,694kcal

5. Male, 30 years old
Height: 177cm (5ft 10in)
Weight: 82kg (180lb)
Occupation: church minister
Event: badminton

Basal rate	1,730kcal
Occupation + chores allowance (=70%)	865kcal
Match play 90min	840kcal
Total (per day)	3,435kcal

6. Male, 19 years old
Height: 177cm (6ft 1in)
Weight: 80kg (175lb)
Occupation: PE student
Event: badminton

Basal rate	1,750kcal
Occupation + chores allowance (=100%)	1,750kcal
Match play 90min	900kcal
Total (per day)	4,400kcal

It is estimated that each game of badminton requires, in terms of energy, approximately 200–280kcal. This, of course, depends upon the size of the player, the level of participation and the duration of the game. The social player fits into the lower part of the limit while the good club player is likely to expend energy closer to the upper limit of the suggested levels.

12

Dietary Considerations for Weight-Lifting and Body-Building

While for convenience I have grouped these two sports together they actually represent two totally different philosophies towards sport. The weight-lifter is concerned with muscle strength and to a degree muscle mass (there is a high correlation between muscle mass and gross strength) in order to lift a very heavy weight. On the other hand, the body-builder is keen to obtain muscle bulk in order to sculpture it into a muscle definition that judges will recognise for its special qualities. However, one only has to be in the company of both types of sportsperson to appreciate that they are committed to their search for excellence and are most aware of the part which nutrition can play in this search.

Like boxing and wrestling, weight-lifting is divided into weight categories where the range is extreme. For example, using the statistics of the 1984 Olympic games weight-lifters, the weight range varied from 51.2kg (113lb) to 152kg (335lb). However, there have been men who have scaled in excess of 160kg (350lb).

Because of the vast difference in size there is a comparable difference in the value of the weights lifted. For example, in the 1980 games the combined total for the snatch and the jerk varied from 245kg (540lb) for the flyweight category to 395kg (870lb) for the super heavyweight.

So, while there is a relationship between physical weight and the competition weight lifted it is not a linear relationship, since skill levels also have a significant effect. For example, again from the 1980 games, the flyweight lifted 245kg (540lb) for a new record, whereas the super heavyweight, whose body-weight was about twice that of the fly-weight, only lifted 395kg (870lb). Had the relationship been linear, the super

Fig 29 Facing page. Judy Oakes who through careful training and eating has largely overcome the handicap of height.

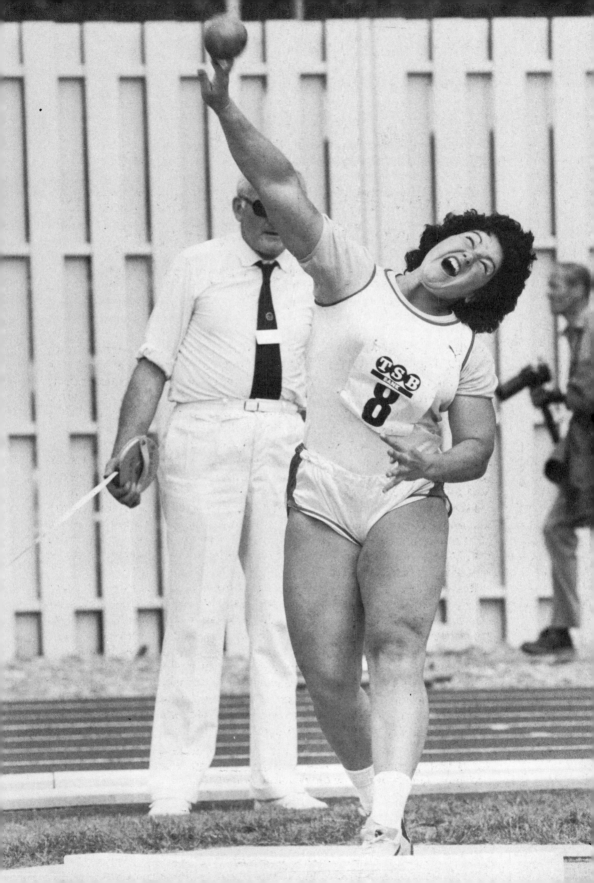

heavyweight should have lifted in excess of 490kg (1,080lb)!

For example, Leonid Zhabotinsky of the Soviet Union snatched 170kg (375lb) for a new record in 1968. He is 184cm (6ft) tall; assuming that the weight went 1m (3ft) above his shoulder height, at full arm's length, the total distance through which the weight moved was 230cm (7ft 6in). With this information it is possible to work out that a lift of this nature would require 80.1kcal in terms of energy. This is possible because of the direct relationship between work and energy so making it quite easy to calculate energy requirements for a single lift. All that is required to be known is the weight of the bar to be lifted and the range through which that weight is lifted. However, because there is such a massive difference in size the basal rate is a very significant (and variable) factor.

Weight category (kg)		Basal rate + chores (kcal/day)	Total energy (kcal/day)
52	Flyweight	2,670	3,970
56	Bantamweight	2,900	4,220
60	Featherweight	3,150	4,510
67.5	Lightweight	3,500	4,900
75	Middleweight	4,000	5,500
82.5	Light heavyweight	4,250	5,850
90	Middle heavyweight	5,000	6,700
110	Heavyweight	5,500	6,900
over 110	Super heavyweight	7,500	9,400

Fig 30   The daily energy requirements of different categories of weight-lifters. These values assume a constant age and a proportional increase in height from one weight category to the next.

Of one thing I am certain: I would not like to have to feed a super heavyweight lifter for any period of time – I have seen the huge amounts of food which they consume at the Olympic games!

The field of nutrition, so far as body-building is concerned, is clouded in mystique, into which I would not care to intrude. One has only to look through the pages of a body-building magazine to realise what a very significant contribution the food-supplement market makes to this sport. I know of one body-builder who spends every penny he earns on food supplements and special food; his current expenditure is well over £100 per week. In this context, it is interesting to note an extract from the training diary of a recent European body-building champion.

Breakfast: 450g (1lb) steamed cod, 2 boiled eggs, herbal tea.

Lunch: one full roast chicken, 1 apple, 2 rye biscuits.

Dinner: 450g (1lb) boiled cod, 450g (1lb) brown rice.

Each meal was followed by supplements of: vitamin C 6g; choline; lecithin; vitamin B_6 and liquid amino acids. In addition there were regular snacks of peanuts, cashew nuts, almonds, fruit and chicken portions. It is interesting to note that there was a total absence of red meat but as this menu was for the pre-competition phase this can be explained by the competitor's desire to restrict the intake of fats. In his training phase several of the meals contained 450g (1lb) beef or lamb.

From a critical point of view the diet might be too low on carbohydrates (although 450g (1lb) rice is a considerable intake) and there is almost a complete absence of vegetables, which could contribute to a vitamin deficiency. However, the snacks could probably compensate for this. I know of several body-builders who take at least one hour each day to take their food supplements alone. These start with 'body-power' break-fast cereal, together with alfalfa, kelp, honey, milk-protein drink, liquid amino acids, choline, inositol, desiccated liver, vitamins B, C and E, multi-mineral and trace element compound, not to mention the non-steroid anabolic pills (a supposedly legal version of the banned drug). All of the supporting literature which accompanies the food supplements give sound physiological reasoning for their use. Because of the sheer cost involved in their diets body-builders must feel good for surely they would not waste their money on ineffective supplements?

Writing in a leading body-building magazine a well-known health-food manufacturer presents the following list of benefits in order to support supplementation. It claims they can:

> enhance the metabolic process of muscle growth
> raise strength levels
> improve aerobic endurance
> reduce body-fat levels
> aid recovery between training sessions
> hasten recovery from injury
> maintain optimum health levels
> reduce pain
> improve concentration

Few enthusiasts could doubt the logic of such a list, which is a supporting argument for their sensible use.

To conclude this section on body-building I would like to present a calculation which begins at the opposite end of the process compared to the others made in this book. Having spent several days in the company of a top-class body-builder I have calculated that his daily food intake (including all snacks) produces an energy equivalent of over 5,000kcal per day. Following this observation up with calliper measurements to calcu- late his percentage of body-fat, it would appear that his energy balance is just right.

13

Proposed Energy Menus

In this chapter I aim to provide suitable, realistic daily menus for all of the energy categories outlined and calculated in Chapters 8–12. They will cover all the various groups, from those who require less than 3,000kcal to those who need in excess of 7,000kcal per day. There is an attempt to include a wide variety of foods – especially those which people actually eat and which are obtainable cheaply. Fresh vegetables and fruit are included in order to help contribute to a healthy diet and to give a good balance of all of the essential nutrients. However, it must be emphasised that it is variety in food which helps to make the most significant contribution to a healthy life. Readers can take parts from all of the diets as long as the total portions add up to the energy category to which individuals belong. But remember that you should monitor your body-weight frequently and then take appropriate steps to make any adjustment which might be necessary.

Part of this chapter will cover the carbohydrate-loading system, as well as making some suggestions for those who might wish to gain or lose weight safely. The diets are intended for use with conventional eating habits (that is three meals a day), which most people involved in sport should try to follow; regular eating habits are important for success. It must be remembered that any snacks or 'social nibbles' must form part of the daily total of energy intake. In every case the amount of each food will be quantified and whenever possible, the appropriate calorific equivalent listed. Again, in every case I have tried to be realistic. I have tended to include foods which I know the best sportspeople eat, especially while away at major competitions. I have lived with such people for extended periods and have come to know their likes and dislikes.

A food which is familiar – and which the person likes – immediately stimulates the digestive system, so making digestion more efficient. Unappetising or badly presented food does very little for this physiological priming. While I have met the odd athlete who has developed an

Breakfast		(kcal)
1 cup cereal with ½ cup full milk, 1tsp sugar		185
2 slices whole-meal toast, low-fat spread, preserve		447
1 cup coffee/tea/herbal tea, white, 1tsp sugar		40
	Total	672
Lunch		
1 salad sandwich		286
1 low-fat yoghurt		89
1 medium apple		159
1pt fresh orange juice		169
	Total	703
Dinner		
150g (5oz) roast chicken		250
2 cups green vegetables		120
1 cup carrots		40
200g (7oz) boiled potatoes		150
4tbsp gravy		45
2 cups rice pudding		405
1 cup coffee/tea/herbal tea, white, 1tsp sugar		40
	Total	1,050
Evening snack		
1 cup warm full milk, plus 1 biscuit		300
	Daily Total	2,725

Fig 31 A menu for 2,500–3,000kcal per day. This example shows a single day.

eccentric pattern of eating too often based on fads rather than proven facts, I have tried to stick to the types of foods usually consumed in the United Kingdom.

The values for the foods are mainly taken from the wrappers or cartons in which they are contained. Where this is not obvious I have used a set of standard tables produced by the World Health Organisation. I must emphasise to readers that without actually measuring the quantity of food eaten on scales an accurate calculation cannot be made. It is not my intention to inflict this scientific approach upon everyone and there may be a margin of error of ten per cent.

In the menus I have tried to permit a very wide variety of food, but at the same time I have had to keep in mind that sport is a very time-consuming exercise and that time spent in shopping and preparation is encroaching upon this valuable time.

In a study of this nature there must be some standard measurements for certain foodstuffs. These are as follows:

a slice of bread from one recognised medium-sliced 450g (1lb) loaf measuring 14 × 10cm (5.1 × 4in)
a standard breakfast cup or glass with a capacity of 0.23l (8fl oz)
the standard measure for teaspoon (tsp) and tablespoon (tbsp)

In order to preserve the value of many nutrients, vegetables should be lightly cooked.

Breakfast		(kcal)
1 glass fresh orange juice		70
75g (3oz) grilled bacon, 1 fried egg, 100g (3½oz)		
grilled tomato		390
2 slices whole-meal toast, low-fat spread, preserve		447
1 cup coffee/tea/herbal tea, white, 1tsp sugar		40
	Total	947
Lunch		
100g (3½oz) cheddar cheese		406
100g (3½oz) mixed green salad		60
100g (3½oz) chipped potatoes		170
1 glass fresh orange juice		169
1 large banana		120
1 cup coffee/tea/herbal tea, white, 1tsp sugar		40
	Total	965
Dinner		
2 cups clear vegetable soup		190
200g (7oz) steak and kidney pie		650
2 cups green vegetables		120
1 cup root vegetables (swede, parsnip, carrot or similar)		120
2 jacket potatoes, 200g (7oz) each		219
4tbsp gravy		400
100g (3½oz) apple pie		370
2tbsp cream		65
Coffee/tea/herbal tea, white, 1tsp sugar		40
	Total	2,174
	Daily Total	**4,086**

Fig 32   A menu for 3,000–4,000kcal per day.

Breakfast		(kcal)
1 glass full milk		160
2 cups cereal, 1 cup full milk, 1tsp sugar		220
100g (3½oz) grilled sausage, 75g (2½oz) grilled bacon		383
1 fried egg		200
100g (3½oz) grilled mushrooms		30
1 slice whole-meal toast, low-fat spread, preserve		220
1 cup coffee/tea/herbal tea, white, 1tsp sugar		40
	Total	1,253
Mid-morning snack		
1 glass full milk		160
1 salad sandwich		220
	Total	380
Lunch		
2 poached eggs on 2 slices of whole-meal toast		550
1 slice chocolate cake, 150g (5oz)		500
1 glass fresh orange juice		220
1 cup coffee/tea/herbal tea, white, 1tsp sugar		40
	Total	1,310
Evening meal		
200g (7oz) poached/grilled fish		420
4tbsp white sauce		86
2 cups mixed green vegetables		120
2 cups mixed root vegetables		120
2 jacket potatoes 200g (7oz) each		219
150g (5oz) tinned peaches/pears		146
100g (3½oz) ice cream		196
2 × 60ml (2fl oz) glasses medium white wine		300
1 cup coffee/tea/herbal tea, white, 1tsp sugar		40
	Total	1,647
Evening snack		
1 cup warm full milk		280
	Daily Total	4,870

Fig 34   A menu for 4,000–5,000kcal per day.

In this section of the book I have tried to indicate what foods can be eaten in order to keep a particular energy balance. The menus should be used as a guide to what is eaten and should stimulate an examination of one's own eating habits.

Breakfast		(kcal)
1pt fresh orange juice		160
1 glass full milk		160
2 cups cereal with full milk, 1tsp sugar		714
100g (3½oz) grilled bacon		238
100g (3½oz) grilled sausage		217
100g (3½oz) grilled tomatoes		15
2 fried eggs		119
3 slices whole-meal toast, low-fat spread, 50g		
(2oz) honey		526
	Total	2,149
Lunch		
2 salad rolls		386
1 low-fat yoghurt		89
1 apple, 1 banana		260
1 glass full milk		160
	Total	895
Mid-afternoon snack		
1 glass full milk		160
1 cheese roll		476
	Total	636
Evening meal		
2 cups oxtail soup		180
200g (7oz) battered fish		397
200g (7oz) chipped potatoes		633
100g (3½oz) peas		26
100g (3½oz) sweet corn		55
200g (7oz) fresh fruit salad		200
200g (7oz) ice cream		309
2 × 60ml (2fl oz) glasses medium white wine		300
1 cup coffee/tea/herbal tea, white, 1tsp sugar		40
	Total	2,140
	Daily Total	5,820

Fig 35   A menu for 5,000–6,000kcal per day.

Special Diets

Very few sports require a special diet. By this I mean that the food eaten by an archer is unlikely to be very different from that of a wrestler. The quantities may differ, as may the preparation, but in basic terms it will still be the same food. In this section, therefore, I will only cover such aspects as carbohydrate loading, weight-loss diets and pre- and post-event diets.

113

Carbohydrate Loading

There are two versions of this diet, both of which are no longer as popular as they were after Saltin first introduced them. The two diets are now termed 'full' or 'partial'. The full uses a period of glycogen depletion whereas the partial uses only the 'loading' aspect. In the full form there are two considerations:

the bleed-out
the loading

In the bleed-out (or depletion) phase the athlete trains hard to deplete the stores of glycogen available in both liver and muscle, while at the same time being starved of carbohydrates through the food intake. This will mean that energy has to be raised from the fat stores and from protein. If, as is likely, the athlete is already thin, the fat stores will be small. Hence protein becomes a primary source of energy. This situation is not without its side-effects, such as the production of urea. According to Saltin, this depletion phase is important since it stimulates the enzymes which bring about the overcompensation effect.

The bleed-out period is usually started at least five days before the planned peak (most athletes use a seven-day approach). The rate at which the energy reserves are depleted depends upon the individual and the intensity of training during the depletion phase. If the training is intense, the depletion period is shortened. However, because of the poorer reserves of energy, training performances during this period are likely to be affected and this frequently has a psychological effect upon the athlete; many report quite serious 'withdrawal' symptoms.

While the term 'starved of carbohydrates' is used during the depletion phase, the body must still have some carbohydrates to supply the nervous system and other vital organs. Once the depletion phase is complete the loading starts. Exercise during this period must be restricted and in fact a complete rest of two days is advocated. Foods rich in carbohydrates should be eaten with a restricted intake of both fats and protein. However, some fats and protein must be taken as they are essential for good health. During this phase fluid intake must be kept high as this also has an effect upon the body's ability to store glycogen.

The theory of carbohydrate loading is wholly dependent upon the ability of the body to overcompensate as a reaction to an imposed stress. In this case the stress is a shortage of glycogen. As a reaction, the body increases its reservoirs of glycogen so making more available for future use. The pattern used by most athletes is one whereby the marathon runner (for example) runs a fast 30km (19m run seven days before a planned peak (usually another important marathon). This starts the depletion phase and is followed by three days of carbohydrate starvation. Three days before the big event loading starts by resting and considerably increasing the intake of carbohydrates.

I know a number of athletes who have used the system and most admit that the disadvantages outweigh the advantages. Several have adopted the partial system, using only a single depletion run much closer to the proposed peak followed by the loading aspect. Some others simply increase their intake of carbohydrates a couple of days before the scheduled race.

It is very important that anyone who proposes to use the Saltin diet should experiment frequently during preparation phases so that he or she becomes familiar with the situation.

Slimming Diets

It is unlikely that any top-class sportsperson will need to slim. Most will have a high energy output to match their energy input. However, I have had to use slimming diets with some athletes, particularly women, who have had a period of absence from training through injury.

The theory of slimming appears at first sight to be a simple one, but it is actually far more complicated, requiring a disciplined approach to two aspects of life; weight can be lost by either reducing the food intake or increasing the energy output. In reality it is the type of food eaten during such a diet which is important.

During attempts to lose weight, fats and other dead calories must be excluded from the diet. Indeed I am in favour of *almost* fasting for two days. I have used the following with a very good degree of success, but it must be stressed that it needs a great deal of self-discipline.

From day 3 it should be possible to follow a diet similar to that listed in this chapter for 2,000–3,000kcal. However, the scales will indicate whether or not this is advisable. The grapefruit in the morning is important because of the enzymic effect it has upon the stomach. Grapes supply the kind of energy needed by the vital organs. It is important to exclude both coffee and tea during this period although other fluid levels must be kept high.

DAY 1

Breakfast
½ fresh grapefruit, 1 cup herbal tea or fruit juice

Lunch
1 cup grapes, 1 cup herbal tea or fruit juice

Dinner
1 boiled egg, 1 slice whole-meal bread and low-fat spread
1 cup herbal tea or fruit juice

DAY 2

Breakfast and lunch
As day 1

Dinner
Grapes, cottage cheese salad

DAY 3

Breakfast
½ fresh grapefruit, 1 slice whole-meal toast, low-fat spread, thin spreading of
preserve

Lunch
Grapes, cottage cheese salad plus low-fat yoghurt, 1 cup herbal tea or fruit juice

Dinner
100g (3½oz) of steamed fish, crunch salad, 1 cup herbal tea or fruit juice

Fig 36   A slimming diet to be rigidly followed.

Pre-Event Meal

It is still not uncommon for competitors from certain sports to go to a restaurant for a pre-match meal. Indeed a club I was associated with, as little as ten years ago, always had a pre-match meal (which included steak) as little as three hours before an important game. This was followed by drinks of sal-volatile on arrival at the ground to make the players sick! Many sportspeople still believe in this very dated and unsound theory of protein before a match. The truth is that this is the last thing needed as the food stays for a long time in the gut, which in turn requires blood for digestion, taking it away from the exercising muscles.

No large meal containing protein should be taken closer than about four hours before a period of contemplated high activity. While it is true to say that the body cannot perform on an 'empty tank' it is equally true to insist that it cannot perform on a very full one. My advice to all sportspeople is to have a very light snack about two hours before an event. My favourite is two slices of whole-meal toast, low-fat spread and honey, together with a drink of sweet, weak tea. This will provide the body with all that it requires. The most important of these at this time is the drink. I know of many athletes who have particular fads, but few of them can be supported by sound nutritional reasoning. However, it is advantageous, particularly before important competitions, for the performer to be relaxed and in as familiar a situation as is possible under such stressful conditions. With such reasoning it is conceivable even to support the ice cream that one outstanding international runner insisted on having one hour before his distance race.

To summarise, the body requires some food and liquid before an event. Simple carbohydrates are the best and one should experiment during preparation phases as to the precise content and timing of this meal. There is no substitute for careful planning and rehearsal. Again, for those events of a longer duration that may require the performer to eat between phases of a competition, the same rules as for pre-event eating apply.

Post-Event Meals

In Chapter 5 the inhibiting effect of exercise upon the appetite was discussed. Here again this should be emphasised; it is most important that the energy replenishment system starts as soon as possible after exercise and this might necessitate a snack of an apple or grapes. After that the performer should allow the natural demands of the body to suggest when it is appropriate to have a meal. This meal should be one rich in carbohydrates; any of those listed earlier in the chapter would be ideal.

Appendix 1

The following table gives energy and nutrient values for a variety of common foods. For the sake of convenience, measurements are given largely in grams and kilocalories. Reference may be made to Appendix 2 for conversion tables from grams to imperial weights and from kilocalories to kilojoules.

	Measure	Approx. weight (g)	Food energy (kcal)	Protein (g)	Fat (g)	Calcium (mg)	Iron (mg)	Vitamin B₁ (mg)	Vitamin B₂ (mg)	Vitamin B₃ (mg)	Vitamin C (mg)
Dairy products											
cow's milk (whole fluid)	1 cup	244	160	9	9	288	0.1	0.07	0.41	0.2	2
cow's milk (non-fat dry)	1 cup	104	375	37	1	1,345	0.6	0.36	1.85	0.9	7
cheddar cheese	1oz.	28	115	7	9	213	0.3	0.01	0.13	trace	—
cottage cheese	1 cup	245	260	33	10	230	0.7	0.07	0.61	0.2	—
processed cheese	1oz.	28	105	7	9	198	0.3	0.01	0.12	trace	—
full cream	1 cup	242	325	8	28	261	0.1	0.07	0.39	0.1	2
ice cream	1 cup	133	255	6	14	194	0.1	0.05	0.28	0.1	1
Eggs											
eggs, medium	each	50	80	6	6	27	1.1	0.05	0.15	trace	—
Meat, poultry, fish											
beef, baked	4oz.	113	326	28	23	12	3.2	0.09	0.24	5.1	—
beef steak, sirloin	4oz.	113	440	24	32	12	3.3	0.06	0.18	4.9	—
pork, grilled	4oz.	113	346	20	28	11	2.8	0.76	0.24	4.6	—
veal	4oz.	113	246	32	12	12	3.0	0.07	0.28	5.3	—
chicken, roasted	4oz.	113	153	25	4	12	1.8	0.07	0.19	8.9	—
haddock/cod, fried	4oz.	113	186	24	6	42	1.3	0.04	0.08	3.2	2
tuna	4oz.	113	226	32	8	9	1.9	0.05	0.13	13.0	—

	Measure	Approx. weight	Food energy	Protein	Fat	Calcium	Iron	Vitamin B$_1$	Vitamin B$_2$	Vitamin B$_3$	Vitamin C
		(g)	(kcal)	(g)	(g)	(mg)	(mg)	(mg)	(mg)	(mg)	(mg)
Dry beans, peas, nuts											
almonds	1 cup	142	850	26	77	332	6.7	0.34	1.31	5.0	trace
beans, dried, cooked	1 cup	180	210	14	1	90	4.9	0.25	0.13	1.3	—
beans, haricot	1 cup	190	260	16	1	55	5.9	0.25	0.11	1.3	—
cashews, roasted	1 cup	140	785	24	64	53	5.3	0.60	0.35	2.5	—
lentils	1 cup	250	265	20	trace	68	5.3	0.93	0.55	5.0	—
peanuts, roasted	1 cup	144	840	37	72	107	3.0	0.46	0.19	24.7	—
peanut butter	1 cup	16	95	4	8	9	0.3	0.02	0.02	2.4	—
peas, dried, cooked	1 cup	250	290	20	1	28	4.2	0.37	0.22	2.2	—
soyabeans, dried, cooked	1 cup	180	208	18	9	117	4.3	0.34	0.14	1.0	—
Vegetables											
asparagus	1 cup	145	30	3	slight	30	0.9	0.23	0.26	2.0	38
beans, green, cooked	1 cup	125	30	2	trace	63	0.8	0.09	0.11	0.6	15
beansprouts, cooked	1 cup	125	35	4	trace	21	1.1	0.11	0.13	0.9	8
beetroot, cooked, sliced	1 cup	170	55	2	trace	24	0.9	0.05	0.07	0.5	10
broccoli, cooked	1 cup	155	40	5	1	136	1.2	0.14	0.31	1.2	140
brussel sprouts, cooked	1 cup	155	55	7	1	50	1.7	0.12	0.22	1.2	135
cabbage, raw	1 cup	70	15	1	trace	34	0.3	0.04	0.04	0.2	33
carrots, raw	each	50	20	1	trace	18	0.4	0.03	0.03	0.3	4
cauliflower, cooked	1 cup	120	25	3	trace	25	0.8	0.11	0.10	0.7	66
celery, large stick	each	40	5	trace	trace	16	0.1	0.01	0.01	0.1	4
corn, sweet, cooked	1 ear	140	70	3	1	2	0.5	0.09	0.08	1.0	7
cucumbers	each	207	30	1	trace	35	0.6	0.07	0.09	0.4	23
lettuce	1 head	454	60	4	trace	91	2.3	0.29	0.27	1.3	29
onions, raw	each	110	40	2	trace	30	0.6	0.04	0.04	0.2	1
parsley	1tbsp.	4	trace	trace	trace	8	0.2	trace	0.01	trace	7
parsnips, cooked	1 cup	155	100	2	1	70	0.9	0.11	0.12	0.2	16
peas, cooked	1 cup	160	115	9	1	37	2.9	0.44	0.17	3.7	33
peppers, sweet	each	74	15	1	trace	7	0.5	0.06	0.06	0.4	94
potatoes, baked, medium	each	99	90	3	trace	9	0.7	0.10	0.04	1.7	20
radishes	each	10	1	trace	trace	3	0.1	trace	trace	trace	2
spinach, cooked	1 cup	108	40	5	1	167	4.0	0.13	0.25	1.0	50
tomatoes	each	200	40	2	trace	24	0.9	0.11	0.07	1.3	42
tomato juice	1 cup	243	45	2	trace	17	2.2	0.12	0.07	1.9	39
turnips	1 cup	155	35	1	trace	54	0.6	0.06	0.08	0.5	34
Fruits and fruit products											
apples, raw	each	150	70	trace	trace	8	0.4	0.04	0.02	0.1	3
apple juice	1 cup	248	120	trace	trace	15	1.5	0.02	0.05	0.2	2
apricots, dried	1 cup	150	390	8	1	100	8.2	0.02	0.23	4.9	19
apricots, tinned	1 cup	251	140	1	trace	23	0.5	0.03	0.03	0.5	8

	Measure	Approx. weight	Food energy	Protein	Fat	Calcium	Iron	Vitamin B_1	Vitamin B_2	Vitamin B_3	Vitamin C
		(g)	(kcal)	(g)	(g)	(mg)	(mg)	(mg)	(mg)	(mg)	(mg)
avocado	each	284	370	5	37	22	1.3	0.24	0.43	3.5	30
banana	each	175	100	1	trace	10	0.8	0.06	0.07	0.8	12
blackberries	1 cup	144	85	2	1	46	1.3	0.05	0.06	0.5	30
dates	1 cup	178	490	4	1	105	5.3	0.16	0.17	3.9	—
figs	each	21	60	1	trace	26	0.6	0.02	0.02	0.1	—
grapefruit	each	482	100	2	trace	40	1.0	0.10	0.04	0.4	88
grapefruit juice	1 cup	247	100	1	trace	20	1.0	0.07	0.04	0.4	84
grapes	1 cup	153	65	1	1	15	0.4	0.05	0.03	0.2	3
lemons	each	110	20	1	trace	19	0.4	0.03	0.01	0.1	39
oranges	each	180	65	1	trace	54	0.5	0.13	0.05	0.5	66
orange juice, fresh	1 cup	248	110	2	1	27	0.5	0.22	0.07	1.0	124
peaches	each	114	35	1	trace	9	0.5	0.02	0.05	1.0	7
pears	each	182	100	1	1	13	0.5	0.04	0.07	0.2	7
pineapple	1 cup	140	75	1	trace	24	0.7	0.12	0.04	0.3	24
plums	each	60	25	trace	trace	7	0.3	0.02	0.02	0.3	3
raisins	1 cup	165	480	4	trace	102	5.8	0.18	0.13	0.8	2
raspberries	1 cup	123	70	1	1	27	1.1	0.04	0.11	1.1	31
strawberries	1 cup	149	55	1	1	31	1.5	0.04	0.10	1.0	88
tangerines	1 cup	116	40	1	trace	34	0.3	0.05	0.02	0.1	27
Sugars, sweets											
honey	1 tbsp.	21	65	trace	—	1	0.1	trace	0.01	0.1	trace
sugar, brown	1 cup	220	280	—	—	187	7.5	0.02	0.07	0.4	—
sugar, white	1 cup	200	770	—	—	—	0.2	—	—	—	—
Grain products											
bread, white	1 lb	454	1,255	39	15	381	11.3	1.13	0.95	10.9	trace
bread, whole-meal	1 lb	454	1,100	48	14	449	13.6	1.18	0.54	12.7	trace
cornmeal, ground	1 cup	122	435	11	5	24	2.9	0.46	0.13	2.4	—
macaroni	1 cup	130	190	6	1	14	1.4	0.23	0.14	1.8	—
oats, rolled	1 cup	240	130	5	2	22	1.4	0.19	0.05	0.2	—
rice, brown, cooked	1 cup	205	238	5	1	24	1.0	0.18	0.04	2.8	—
rice, white, cooked	1 cup	205	225	4	trace	21	1.8	0.23	0.02	2.1	—
white flour	1 cup	120	400	16	2	49	4.0	0.66	0.14	5.2	—
whole-wheat flour	1 cup	115	420	12	1	18	3.3	0.51	0.30	4.0	—
Fats and oils											
butter	½ cup	113	810	1	92	23	—	—	—	—	—
cooking fats:											
lard/dripping	1 cup	205	1,850	—	205	—	—	—	—	—	—
vegetable fats	1 cup	200	1,770	—	200	—	—	—	—	—	—
margarine	½ cup	113	815	1	92	23	—	—	—	—	—
oils, sunflower etc.	1 cup	220	1,945	—	220	—	—	—	—	—	—

Appendix 2

Conversion Tables

Weight

g (grams)	oz. (ounces)
1	0.04
2	0.07
3	0.11
4	0.14
5	0.18
6	0.21
7	0.25
8	0.28
9	0.32
10	0.35
20	0.71
30	1.06
40	1.41
50	1.76
60	2.12
70	2.47
80	2.82
90	3.17
100	3.53
200	7.06
300	10.6
400	14.1
500	17.6
600	21.2
700	24.7
800	28.2
900	31.8
1000	35.3

Energy

kilocalories (kcal)	kilojoules (kJ)
1	4.18
2	8.37
3	12.6
4	16.7
5	20.9
6	25.1
7	29.3
8	33.5
9	37.7
10	41.8
20	83.7
30	126
40	167
50	209
60	251
70	293
80	335
90	377
100	418
200	837
300	1260
400	1670
500	2090
600	2510
700	2930
800	3350
900	3770
1000	4180

Glossary

Adipose tissue Fat cells which are stored about the body. They are necessary for cosmetic, thermal and energy-production reasons. An excess produces obesity.

ADP and ATP ATP (adenosine triphosphate) is the chemical material which gives the muscle cells energy to contract. Once it has been used a phosphate is lost and it becomes ADP (adenosine diphosphate). When it is 'given' a phosphate from phosphocreatine (PC) ATP is re-formed to keep the energy cycle continuous.

Aerobic Combustion with sufficient oxygen.

Alfalfa A plant of the lucerne family.

Alkali An alkali neutralises an acid.

Amenorrhoea The arresting of the menstrual cycle, a condition common among those women who have reduced body-fat levels.

Amino acid The form in which protein is available in the body.

Anabolic Building-up, hence anabolic steroids which promote muscle growth.

Anaemia A condition in which there is a reduced level of red blood-cells necessary for the transportation of oxygen.

Anaerobic Combustion without oxygen.

Anorexia The loss of appetite, frequently a psychological disorder. Unless arrested it is certain to produce death.

Basal rate The basic rate of the metabolism, for example during bed rest.

Biomechanics The laws of physics applied to human motion.

Biotin A B-group vitamin.

Blood buffers A store of alkaline substances which can neutralise the blood if it is too acidic.

Calciferol A form of the sunlight-dependent vitamin D.

Calcium An essential mineral which aids bone and teeth growth.

Calorie A unit of heat applied here to the capacity of foods to produce energy. Although strictly speaking foods are usually measured in thousands of calories – kilocalories – as in this book, common usage erroneously has calories.

Calorimeter An instrument used in experiments to measure heat, for example, the Bomb calorimeter used in the determination of the calorific value of foods.

Carbohydrate A compound made up of carbon, hydrogen and oxygen. A good provider of energy.

Carbohydrate loading A method for improving one's potential store of energy.

Cardiac Pertaining to the heart, for example the cardiac muscle is the heart muscle.

Carnitine An amino acid.

Catalyst A substance which makes a chemical reaction more efficient without a change in its own basic structure.

Cellular fluid The life-giving fluid in which all cells are bathed.

Cholesterol A substance similar to alcohol manufactured in the body, which can increase the likelihood of heart disease.

Choline A B group vitamin.

Chyme The acid state of the food before digestion occurs.

CNS The central nervous system, the communication network of the body.

CORI-cycle The sequence of events in which lactic acid is re-formed into glycogen by the liver and delivered back into the bloodstream.

Coronary Artery and vein. The vessels that deliver blood directly to and from the heart muscle.

Creatine phosphate (phosphocreatine, PC) A substance stored in the body allowing the completion of the ATP and ADP cycle to provide energy.

Degrade To break down.

Dehydration Shortage of fluid, as in high-level exercise in hot, humid conditions. Body fluid is lost in an attempt to keep the core temperature stable.

Depressant Something which will have a depressing, steadying, slowing effect.

Dietary fibre A vegetable foodstuff which is not totally broken down during digestion. It passes through the digestive tract taking with it toxic products.

Disaccharides A combination of two simple sugars, for example sucrose.

Duodenum The part of the digestive tract immediately following the stomach.

Dynamics The branch of physics which deals with movement.

Electrolyte Salts or ions dissolved in body fluid which can be electrically charged (either positive or negative).

123

Endocrine   A ductless gland which produces hormones.

Energy   The potential to do work. Energy is transferred from one source to another, the primary source being the sun.

Enzyme   A protein molecule that makes chemical reactions in the body more efficient.

Ergogenic   Pertaining to work.

Extent of loading   A term used in training theory to describe the quantity of work.

Ferrograd C   An iron fumerate preparation containing vitamin C to aid absorption of the iron.

Folic acid   A member of the B group of vitamins.

Force   A term used in physics – that which will change the state of a body at rest or its uniform motion in a straight line.

Fructose   A single sugar (monosaccharide), found in fruit, especially grapes. Combines with glucose to make sucrose.

Galactose   A single sugar (monosaccharide), which combines with glucose to make lactose.

Gall-bladder   The organ which stores bile (secreted into the duodenum during digestion).

Glutamine and glutamic acid   Amino acids important in the purification process.

Glycerol   A component of the fatty acid triglycerol.

Glycine   An amino acid.

Glycogen   The stored form of glucose energy.

Glycolysis   The breakdown of carbohydrates to form molecules of ATP.

Haemoglobin   The iron pigment in the red blood-cell capable of transporting oxygen.

HCG   Human chorionic gonadotrophin – a growth hormone.

Homoeostasis   The balancing effect of all the body functions, which keeps the internal environment constant.

Hormone   A chemical secreted by the endocrine system. Together with the CNS it brings about homoeostasis.

Inositol   A member of the vitamin B group.

Insulin   A hormone which controls blood-sugar level.

Intensity   A term of training theory used to quantify the pressure or loading.

Intermittent   Used here to describe a form of training in which bouts of exercise are interspersed with rest periods.

Intestine   The region of the alimentary canal from which most of the nutrients are absorbed.

Iodine   An element which influences the thyroid gland.

Joule (J)   The new standard unit of energy; 1cal = 4.184 J (so 1kcal = 4.184kJ).

Kilocalorie (kcal)   One thousand calories.

Lactic acid   An acid produced during respiration and energy utilisation of a high level.

Lecithin   A phospho-lipid, found particularly in coating of nervous tissue.

Leucine   An essential amino acid.

Lipids   Fats or similar substances.

Lysine   An essential amino acid.

Magnesium   An essential mineral which acts as a co-enzyme in producing ATP.

Manganese   An essential mineral with a key function in regulating blood-sugar levels.

Metabolism   The process of turning nutrients into living matter.

Methionine   An essential amino acid.

Microgram   One thousandth of a milligram (one millionth of a gram).

Milligram   One thousandth of a gram.

Mitochondria   Specialised structure within cells associated with the release of ATP.

Molecule   The smallest particle of matter which can exist alone.

Monosaccharide   A single sugar.

Morphology   The study of the form or shape of plants and animals.

Nicotinic acid   Niacin (vitamin B_3).

Oesophagus   The gullet, the canal leading from the mouth to the stomach.

Ornithine   A non-essential amino acid.

Osmosis   Fluid transfer through a membrane.

Oxidation   The addition of oxygen, especially during combustion in order to produce energy.

Pancreas   An organ situated just behind the stomach which secretes digestive juices into the tract.

Pangamic acid   Vitamin B_{15}.

Pantothenic acid   A B-group vitamin, essential for growth.

Parkinson's disease   A disease of the nervous system with an associated tremor.

Peristalsis   A vibratory type of movement which forces food along the digestive pathways.

Phenyalanine   An essential amino acid.

Physics   The science of matter and energy.

Physiology   The study of living organisms.

Phosphogens   High-energy compounds.

Phospho-lipid   A combination of phosphate and glycerol.

Photosynthesis   A process whereby green plants make carbohydrates using carbon dioxide and giving off oxygen.

PMT   Pre-menstrual tension – a condition experienced by some adult women before their monthly periods.

Probenicid   A drug used in the treatment of gout, which also serves as a 'blocking' agent to disguise the presence of other drugs in the urine.

Proline   A non-essential amino acid.

Prostaglandin   A fatty acid which causes contraction of muscles.

Pyridoxine   Vitamin B_6.

Pyruvic acid   A by-product of the aerobic combustion of carbohydrates.

Riboflavin   Vitamin B_2.

Selenium   A water-soluble non-metallic element.

Sodium   A metallic element found only in a combined state in nature, for example sodium chloride (salt).

Steroids   A large group of organic compounds including some hormones.

Taurine   A non-essential amino acid.

Thermodynamics   The study of heat and energy.

Thiamine   Vitamin B_1.

Threonine   An essential amino acid.

Trace elements   Essential minerals required by the body in very small amounts.

Tranquiliser   A drug which brings about a tranquil state and diminishes anxiety.

Triglyceride   The form in which fat is mainly stored in the body (it is a combination of glycerol and fatty acids).

Tryptophan   An essential amino acid.

Tyrosine   A non-essential amino acid.

Valine   An essential amino acid.

Vasodilator   A drug which dilates blood capillaries, so increasing the flow of blood.

$\dot{V}O_2$max   A measure of one's oxygen carrying potential.

Zinc   A metallic element – an essential mineral for the body.

Index